A WORD TO THE WISE

A WORD TO THE WISE
Don Quixote Returns to Fight Perversion

Françoise Davoine and
Jean-Max Gaudillière

Translated by Agnès Jacob

Routledge
Taylor & Francis Group
LONDON AND NEW YORK

First published in English 2018
by Routledge
2 Park Square, Milton Park, Abingdon, Oxon OX14 4RN

and by Routledge
711 Third Avenue, New York, NY 10017

Routledge is an imprint of the Taylor & Francis Group, an informa business

Originally published in French as *A bon entendeur, salut! Face à la perversion, le retour de Don Quichotte* by Stock in 2013.

British Library Cataloguing-in-Publication Data
A catalogue record for this book is available from the British Library

Library of Congress Cataloging-in-Publication Data
A catalog record has been requested for this book

ISBN: 978-1-78220-622-4 (pbk)

Typeset in Palatino LT Std
by Medlar Publishing Solutions Pvt Ltd, India

La depravada edad nuestra

Our depraved era

Don Quixote,
Volume II,
chapter 1, p. 405

CONTENTS

ACKNOWLEDGEMENTS

This book was inspired by lectures given at the École des hautes études en sciences sociales (School of Social Sciences): "The Political Consequences of Trauma", 2000 to 2001; and "The Deaths of Don Quixote", 2002 to 2003. We are grateful to all the participants.

ABOUT THE AUTHORS

Françoise Davoine obtained an *Agregation* in classics (French literature, Latin and Greek) in 1966, followed by a doctorate in sociology in 1981, before becoming a psychoanalyst. She worked for thirty years as a psychoanalyst in public psychiatric hospitals in France, and as an external consultant and is currently in private practice. She was a Professor at the Centre for the Study of Social Movements, École des Hautes Études en Sciences Sociales (EHESS) in Paris, where she and Jean-Max Gaudillière conducted a weekly seminar on "Madness and the Social Link". She has also made numerous presentations at the Austen Riggs Center in Massachusetts (USA), as well as elsewhere in the US, in England, Sweden, Finland, Greece, Mexico, Brazil, Argentina, and Switzerland. Dr Davoine is the author of many articles and books, including *La Folie Wittgenstein*, *Mother Folly*, and *History Beyond Trauma* (with Jean Max Gaudillière).

Jean-Max Gaudillière became a psychoanalyst and member of the Ecole Freudienne in Paris when he discovered the impact of the historical catastrophies reflected in the symptoms of patients confined to asylums. In the weekly seminar called "Madness and the Social Link", held for forty years at the EHESS with Françoise Davoine, Gaudillière combined his clinical work with the exploration of literary works dealing with the madness of war, written by authors like Kenzaburo Oe, Tonni Morrison, Strindberg, Feydeau, Pat Barker, Bion, Musil, Rabelais, Kerouac and Kurt Vonnegut and others. He often referred to the Greek authors of antiquity, whose work he knew intimately. He published numerous articles and gave many conferences. A member of the ISPS US and Erikson Scholar at Austen Riggs Center, he is the co-author of two books written with Françoise Davoine: *History Beyond Trauma* and *A Word to the Wise*. He died in March 2015.

CHAPTER ONE

The child rebels

The return of Don Quixote

All is well. At last we can live in peace, enjoy life! World wars are over, slavery and totalitarian systems have been abolished; all that is in thc past.

At the turn of the seventeenth century, Cervantes is almost ready to believe this. Now that he is over sixty and has gained fame throughout Europe, America, and as far as China, he can devote himself to more noble works than his *Don Quixote*.

But, once again, something goes awry. He must start over, return to the Preface, in which he confesses to a friend that he is in low spirits. What happened? An appalling sequel to the knight's adventures has just been published, written by a swindler attempting to profit from the book's popularity. The counterfeit novel is published under an alias (Canavaggio, 1991). Cervantes calls the author an impostor straight away. Still, he cannot avoid some soul-searching.

If I were him, I would regret having subjected my son, Don Quixote, to the shame of being placed in a cage at the end of the first novel, and of being kidnapped, in chapter XLVI (De Cervantes, 1605/1615), by his own masked friends, who ambush him in his sleep and lock him in a cage.

I would regret having laughed with them at the pathetic puppet carried home on an ox cart. Now, Cervantes gets his just rewards. His novel, whose fame has spread far and wide, and of which over twelve thousand copies have been printed (De Cervantes, 1605/1615, p. 415), is kidnapped in its turn by a literary rascal who "hides his name and disguises his country". To this day, the true identity of Avellaneda, native of Tordesillas, remains unknown.

Passed down from father to son, abduction is re-enacted. More than thirty years after Cervantes' capture by Barbary pirates in 1575, his offspring is captured by other barbarians, from cultured circles this time, less exotic than the Algerian pirates.

"Intergenerational transmission of trauma!" declares the twenty-first century reader. For my part, I had imagined that Cervantes' traumas had been overcome thanks to the psychotherapy conducted by Don Quixote, who undertakes to fight his author's melancholia. I had argued that through his madness, the knight becomes a true psychoanalyst (Davoine, 2016). Could I have been mistaken? I can just hear the chorus of the experts. Of course it is not psychoanalysis! It's definitely not sociology, say the sociologists of my School. Neither is this book suitable for the market, publishers reckon. "You are not my daughter", my mother used to say. Something must be wrong.

In truth, Cervantes is no kinder to his son. In the Preface, he describes the knight as "whimsical [...], full of thoughts of all sorts and such as never came into any other imagination"; consequently, he prefers to declare himself Don Quixote's stepfather, rather than his father (De Cervantes, 1605/1615, p. 3). A hint of cruelty slipped into this declaration of paternity. "I was often cruel to you", my mother confessed at the end of her life. I thought it best not to reply.

Hubris: she's too much!

All-powerful in regard to his creation, has Cervantes sinned by self-love? Or by *hubris*, an offence that the gods of Antiquity could not abide? Has his worldwide fame blinded him to the point where he can let his knight appear in an abject novel?

"Don't put on airs", my grandmother used to say, to save me from such a dreadful fate. And yet she had not read Ovid's *Metamorphoses* (AD 8). But Cervantes had. He knew by heart these stories of catatonic young girls turned into trees, flowers, rivers, or rocks, to escape the violent desires of the gods, and especially their fury when mortals dared to compete with them.

Thus, Psyche—our soul, in Greek, without whom psychoanalysis would not even exist—becomes as mad as our Knight of the Sorrowful Countenance, literally Eroto-maniac, to escape the wrath of Venus, who has sworn to kill her. Her story is recounted in another metamorphosis, *The Golden Ass* (1999), written a century and a half later by the North African writer Apuleius. Psyche offended Venus by being too beautiful. The beauty of her intelligence inspired even greater envy.

Don Quixote is not handsome but is far from stupid. At the end of his novel, Cervantes subjects him to the mockery of bystanders, ignoring his hero's most basic needs, and, above all, disregarding his work of "knight-errantry" (De Cervantes, 1605/1615, p. 384), which made it possible to record the true story of Cervantes' battles and his years of slavery in Algiers. What an ungrateful wretch! Worse still, he is ashamed of his offspring; before abandoning him at the end of the novel—for good, as far as he knows—he lets him know: "You are not my son."

Considered to have written the precursor of the modern novel, does Cervantes predict our current veneration of the ego? I don't think so. And yet, his attitude towards his son brings to mind the injunctions in great vogue today: enjoying oneself, thinking of one's needs, taking care of oneself, having a good self-image, starting a new life in our old age, to be more trendy, less contemptible. Encouraged by his belated literary success, Cervantes now writes incessantly: plays, *Exemplary Stories*, and sea adventures, to woo other maidens under cooler skies than the stifling expanses of La Mancha.

Now that I too have reached the age of white-haired discernment, I dare to say that Cervantes deserves what happened to him. Despite his four centuries of international success, I find it unforgivable that he betrayed his son and had him confined. Nowadays the knight would not escape the standard treatments: electroshock, repeated injections, isolation room—all reported to me daily by former violated children, "full of thoughts […] such as never came into any other imagination", who went berserk in adolescence and were then exposed to chemical and electrical humiliations for over twenty years, sometimes with the complicity of psychoanalysis.

This is why, at the risk of not being considered an analyst or a sociologist, a writer or even my mother's daughter, I dare to inform posterity about a case of abuse perpetrated against the son of the "one-armed man of Lepanto", who turned him into "a brute beast" (De Cervantes, 1605/1615, p. 404), as Cervantes confessed when he finally wrote the true sequel to the knight's adventures, to do him justice.

Do synapses have a soul?

In the meantime, having become the icon his father wished him to be, Don Quixote is also about to lose his soul in the deal set up around him.

"Soul"—a word now out of date in psychotherapeutic circles, for mental illness takes up all the room and no one thinks of the soul any more. Cervantes didn't either. Condemned to house arrest, Don Quixote "eyed them askance, and could not make out where he was" (De Cervantes, 1605/1615, p. 387); Cervantes concluded that nothing more could be done. Freud probably made no objection either. After his early infatuation with the knight during his youth, he may have considered that his psychosis was not amenable to transference. Therefore, he left him behind, preferring the nobler Oedipus, at once more tragic and more theatrical. What an injustice!

And yet, Don Quixote has proven his skill as an analyst with Cardenio, the madman of the Sierra Morena (De Cervantes, 1605/1615, p. 154). Of course, he breaks down later in the novel, but what of it? These things happen! Is it a reason to consider his psychosis incurable, especially after having exploited his psychic energy? Well, Cervantes prescribes him a healthy diet of "good things to eat; [...] for all this madness [...] comes of having the stomach empty and the brains full of wind" (De Cervantes, 1605/1615, p. 404). Still, he endorses the age-old concept of a psychotic structure combined with a brain defect. From there, it is easy to predict a genetic fate, as was already the custom in the Middle Ages, although at the time it was also said that "Insanity is more a tool than a destiny" (in French: *la folie est plus engin que destin*) (De Rotelande, c. 1180). In the end, Cervantes adopts this psychodynamic definition to recover the knight's ingeniousness and reclaim his psyche, held hostage by morons.

That's fortunate, because today the psychoanalytic community, just as Psyche's entourage, would abandon her on her cliff, to expose her to microscopes and cameras that would probe and pursue her, without ever finding her, in the folds of her brain. Terrified, as if caught in a fly trap, she knocks against the cranial wall and collides with dead-end diagnoses, not knowing what is happening, held prisoner by the limits of language.

But "language is not a cage!" objects the knight's admirer, Ludwig Wittgenstein (1929). "When the toolbox with the names is broken" (Wittgenstein, 1953), what cannot be said can always be shown! But can Psyche take note of this language game?

Alas, Psyche has become too human! She is perpetually guilt-ridden since she has been hoisted to the top of the hierarchy of the living, as if nature itself depended on her. No sooner has she survived the totalitarian regimes of the last century, than she accepts the blame for climate change. She is responsible for global warming and for the depletion of energy resources, not only physical, but also economic and psychic.

Morale is low. Earthquakes and upheavals spoil our wonderful beaches, and floods interface with our travels to exotic destinations, killing countless natives at the same time. Then, a volcano awakens just in time to spoil our next vacation. Psyche starts to lose sleep and gulps down all kinds of substances which stimulate financial markets but end up plunging her into depression after each peak of excitement when she thought she was contributing to the greater good.

She no longer knows where to turn, or even where her home is. Like Don Quixote, she has been taken hostage by faceless imposters who stuff her with degraded slogans and recycled drugs sold even to children to keep them quiet. Should we forget about her? She looks so old, poor Psyche! She has put on so much weight that it's hard to recognise her.

Stand up and speak

Indeed, now that I have reached the age at which Cervantes fell prey to swindlers, I can stand up and speak, just as a quarter of a century ago Sarah Smith, an Iroquois potter living on Manitoulin Island in Ontario, predicted that I would do.

In effect, when I encounter in my office a person with a distressed psyche and a downcast gaze, who has nothing to say—there is no use—I see myself standing up and speaking, even while remaining seated. Sometimes, other analysts tell me that they do the same thing, adding: "It's not psychoanalysis, is it?"

So what impels us to take the lead and make contact with people who are hopeless as candidates for psychoanalysis? Ordinarily, transference should proceed in the other direction.

Indeed, we find ourselves in a topsy-turvy world: that of fools, the Innocent, and children whose feast, in Cervantes' era, was celebrated on the same day, 28 December. In fact, an analyst ready to confront madness is often impelled to take on this task by the child he once was, and who witnessed the kidnapping of Psyche through distortions of the truth. Lacking human interlocutors, these old children know how to speak to the soul of things, of plants or of Rocinantes. They all speak to them. "All is sentient", says Nerval (1854). But when they think that they alone see, sense, and hear, they take fright and are said to be delusional.

"More a tool than a destiny"; Folly can, thanks to such reversed transferences, change a destiny in which Psyche is condemned to wither away. To prevent such a fate, Cervantes finally forces himself to leave the desk at which he sits writing other masterpieces, and go visit his confined son. What words did they exchange? In any case, in the Second Part of the adventures, Don Quixote's madness becomes a weapon serving to combat perversion, after having been used in the First Part to free the author from his post-traumatic stress disorder.

When he gets back into action, Cervantes declares—speaking of the author of the false *Don Quixote*, in the Preface of the Second Part—"with his bread let him eat it". And he proceeds to call back Don Quixote, whom he himself has contributed to confine *ad vitam eternam*.

Animism: regenerating the soul

But what can be done to rekindle the spark of Don Quixote's Psyche? Cervantes starts by appealing to the child who loved books of chivalry and was "fond of reading even the very scraps of paper in the streets". Then he sets his son loose in the space of five hundred new pages, with the avowed purpose of having him die, so that no one can kidnap him this time.

At last, Cervantes hears what his son has never tired of claiming, until he was reduced to silence by being forced into disability leave. Catastrophes are his speciality: reinstating the given word, and the honour of widows, orphans, and maidens who go "as spotless virgins to the grave as the mothers that bore them", not only in turbulent times, but also in the face of the corruption encountered in peacetime.

The first novel proved that the sphere of trauma contains huge reserves of energy which, when filtered bit by bit in the course of various adventures, restore us through cathartic processes known the world over. In all periods of human history, in all parts of the earth except, perhaps, in our overly enlightened societies, a soldier returning from combat—or his descendants when the father is not up to the task—must go through a transition ritual to wash away the stain of spilled blood and treat his wounded soul, as well as those of his relatives.

"Man is a ceremonial animal", Wittgenstein (1967) tells us. Cervantes follows this principle. In the first *Don Quixote*, he reinvents the social link for the one who stared death in the face. Ceremonial theatre gave us Eschyles, a veteran of the Greco-Persian War, as well as Sophocles who, at the age of sixteen, conducted the chorus of victory after the battle of Salamin, before being elected general twice in the battle against Samos. The aim of these tragedians was to restore the psyche of their fellow citizens, who were required to attend the plays. Socrates himself fought several wars, to which Alcibiades bears witness at the end of the *Symposium* (Plato, c. 385–370 BC). To the same end, North American Indian societies use ritual masks that the Iroquois of Ontario call "false faces".

During a pow-wow on the plains of South Dakota, and on the Wikwemikong Reservation in Ontario, which I visited in the summer of 1983, everyone stands up when a feather drops to the ground. Among those present at the ceremony, there were few pale faces. Wearing feather headdresses or military berets decorated with medals, veterans of the two World Wars, Korea, and Vietnam danced to the sound of drums and the rhythm of chants, while a feather slowly descended, to honour the soul of fallen companions.

I had the impression of seeing the descent of the winged soul in Plato's *Phaedrus* (c. 370 BC), when it falls out of its chariot drawn by two steeds pulling in opposite directions. Of course, Psyche is not left unscathed, and "her wings fall from her". Socrates speaks of madness (*mania*), brought on by visions (*eideia*) received before the fall, when the souls follow the chariots of an array of gods, circling around the real (*to on*). Did the Ojibwe soul follow the procession of Ares, the god of war? As for Don Quixote, he declares that "chivalry is a religion" (De Cervantes, 1605/1615, p. 444).

As a true medicine man and son of a midwife, Socrates recommends to the one who "is truly possessed and duly out of his mind (*tô orthôs manenti*) [to transform] the wrath (*menis*) [...] transmitted through some lignage (*genos*) into ceremonies (*telestai*), and [...] inspired utterances" (Plato, c. 370 BC). Thus, this veritable analysis of the psyche can beget the art of augury (*mantike*). Socrates points out that it suffices to add to *manike*, meaning mad, the "t" of history (*istoria*), to create the adjective "prophetic" (*mantike*), referring to the gift of divination.

In the Second Part of *Don Quixote*, the hero declares that his own psyche also followed Apollo's chariot, and transformed his madness into poetry, in the tradition of "poets [...] also called *vates*, that is to say diviners" (De Cervantes, 1605/1615, p. 408). Here, we have a remedy to planetary exhaustion. In all eras, everywhere, ceremonial language games continue to transform the deadly impact of traumas into visual, architectural, melodic, rhythmic, poetic, epic, and narrative surviving forms, which are part of humankind's heritage.

Son of a bitch

Yet Cervantes still has a problem. The first *Don Quixote* did indeed bring about a catharsis applauded by European readers and beyond. But another trauma has occurred, an attempted soul murder worse than an attack by pirates, since it is perpetrated within his own camp. Despite his purported indifference regarding the identity of the forger, the mystery intrigues him.

Is the writer of the counterfeit novel the soldier and author Jeronimo de Pasamonte, barely disguised in the first book as Gines de Pasamonte, whom Cervantes has already called "son of a bitch" through the voice of Don Quixote? (De Cervantes, 1605/1615, p. 143). What did this man do to deserve the insult? In the First Part, we learn that Gines was the only one who went to the galleys willingly, planning to write the story of his life during the long winter months, like the true *picaro* he was, fond of knavery. But Cervantes, who has been through many a struggle, cannot bear to see the fascination exerted by this man posing as a rebel. In response to Don Quixote's question about the book he is writing, *The Life of Gines de Pasamonte*, the latter answers loftily: "How can it be finished, when my life is not yet finished?" (De Cervantes, 1605/1615, p. 143). And he adds that the book is already profitable, although he himself has not yet been freed.

Cervantes despises predatory and anti-cathartic literature which traps the reader in areas of death on the pretext of remaining realistic. Inscribing traumas in the memory does not consist in gluing the reader to them, but rather in linking him to myths and spirits of nature, which the knight invokes constantly in order to draw upon their demonic energy. Unable to attain such spheres, Gines is guilty of betraying poetry, in the knight's opinion. Pasamonte's only talent is to provide the reader with an excursion through a world of crime in which he plays the role of gang leader. Later, Cervantes will bring him back on the scene as a puppet showman, braggart, and exploiter of other people's desires (De Cervantes, 1605/1615, p. 542).

True to his nature, the counterfeiter also manipulates Cervantian characters as if they were puppets. He cuts them off from the soul of their "favourite things"—sung by Julie Andrews (Roggers and Hammerstein, 1965) and reinterpreted by John Coltrane in his famous extended version—to which they are attached, life-giving things ensuring survival. In Sioux ceremonies, each participant in turn invokes "all my relatives", not only family members, but also animals, trees, or rocks, for man is located at the bottom of the hierarchy of beings; this is why those who are "duly out of their minds", are right to speak to trees, insects, dogs, the moon, the birds, horses, and donkeys when human beings fail them.

> Free-thinker, Man, do you think you alone
> Think, while life explodes everywhere?
> Respect an active spirit in the creature:
> Each flower is a soul open to Nature;
> In metal a mystery of love is sleeping;
> "All is sentient!" Has power over your being.

Is Cervantes an animist? Like the "Golden Lines" in Nerval's *Chimeras* (1854), inspired by Pythagoras, his two novels link us to the cathartic tradition with its proven symbolic efficiency. Freud, his disciple, also drew upon this tradition.

Freud and Aby Warburg

A little over a century ago, Freud invented psychoanalysis by modernising catharsis to make it science-worthy. In 1895, taking the physics of his time as a model, he wrote his *Project for a Scientific Psychology*. Today considered outdated by science, Freud suffers the same fate as Cervantes. Psychoanalysis has been taken hostage by imbeciles. Who is to blame? After having loved the knight madly—so much that he learned Spanish to read Cervantes in the original—Freud left Don Quixote behind, turning away from madness and trauma. As a result, Quixotic psyches are left in the hands of the same barbers and curates who imprisoned the knight.

And yet, the admirer of Cervantes had recognised the energy emanating from the unnamable and irrepresentable Real, which he named "Omega". At work in the symptoms of trauma and in delusions, it resembles the toxic power of the gods when they make mortals their prey. This is why the *Project* describes the psychic apparatus as a reprocessing plant, using a series of filters, in which Psyche is in charge of sorting. How does she go about it?

Through the first "filtering" of the primary process, called "phi" (Lacan, 1997, Book VII), a senseless energy is channelled into forms Freud calls "thing/word representations". His contemporary, Aby Warburg, describes them as "surviving forms, *nachleben*", or *pathos formel*, saturated with energy, on which he focuses his enquiry, both scientific and psychotic. In 1914, he was raving that he was conducting the war, but he never dissociated his delusions from his research in the field of Renaissance art history. He resolutely refused to be medicated and treated like a case, so that he could continue to think.

When the war ended, he was hospitalised in Switzerland by his brothers, who were Hamburg and US bankers; there, in the Binswanger clinic, he would scream every morning that he was in hell, that all Jews would be exterminated, and that he was being fed human flesh. His psychiatrist, Ludwig Binswanger, was the head perpetrator of these "crimes" at the picturesque Bellevue clinic located on the banks of Lake Constance.

In fact, the German Minister of Foreign Affairs, Walther Rathenau, who was a Jew and a friend of his older brother Max, would be assassinated soon afterwards, in 1922, by right-wing extremists. Tired of fighting with his patient, the famous doctor Binswanger, a Freud disciple, promised Warburg he would discharge him in the highly unlikely event that he would be able to present his research for one hour to an audience composed of the clinic staff and patients.

"I do not believe that *quo ante* recovery from acute psychosis is possible, any more than a return to his scientific activities", Binswanger wrote in a letter addressed to Freud in November 1921, displaying the usual double language of hope held out to the patient on the one hand, and the hopelessness recorded in his files (Warburg, 1923a, p. 14). But Aby took him at his word and decided to disprove the pessimistic prognosis. The challenge to which he responded gave us the famous "Lecture on Serpent Ritual of Hopi Indians", which he presented on 21 April 1923.

In it, he put all his energy into demonstrating how man can give voice to the "seismograph of the soul" (Warburg, 1938–1939, pp. 52–53).

This unconscious device records images that survive the process of denial. Very different from the unconscious related to repressed material, which resorts to signifiers, this seismograph works when language fails. When he delivered his lecture, Aby succeeded in bringing about his own catharsis by linking Renaissance art to the animist rites of Ancient Greece, through the "living archeology" of the rituals of the New Mexico Indian tribes he visited thirty years earlier, on the occasion of the wedding of two of his brothers in the United States.

During the ritual he describes, the Hopi Indians dance for half an hour while holding dangerous rattlesnakes in their mouths. Afterwards, they release them into the desert where, in their crevices in the ground, they are in contact with the ancestors and rekindle psychic energy as well as fertilising rainstorms. In his conclusion, Warburg wrote: "What we have seen in this all too brief summary of the snake cult is intended to show the change from real and substantial symbolism which appropriates by actual gestures to that symbolism which exists in thought alone" (Warburg, 1939, pp. 277–292).

That day, the historian took hold of the *daimons* of his madness. He was able to bear witness for his audience of their link with animist traditions, using the "association of practices recommended by his contemporary Ludwig Wittgenstein, on the model of association of ideas in psychoanalysis". Don Quixote's visit to the cave of Montesinos was soon to illustrate the same method of regeneration.

Binswanger kept his word and released his patient, taking advantage of this therapeutic success to advertise his clinic. But in truth, there is no evidence that he was himself Aby's analyst. On the other hand, the historian had the unwavering support of his young disciple, Fritz Saxl (Binswanger, 2007), who brought him books each time he visited, even during his delusional episodes. Thanks to the transference of this *therapon* (Nagy, 1979), his second in combat—a true Sancho Panza—Aby was able to "exorcise death, put death to death through the symbolism of language", as Wittgenstein says.

Both Warburg and Wittgenstein strongly opposed objectification in the human sciences. Aby Warburg screamed that he refused to be treated like a case (1939), and Wittgenstein wrote: "Frazer is much more savage than most of his savages [...]. His explanations of primitive practices are much cruder than the meaning of these practices themselves" (1967).

The second finer filtering described by Freud in the *Project*, designated as the secondary process, "psi", consists of signifiers, plays on words, which constitute the repressed unconscious and trigger our dreams, parapraxes, and slips of the tongue. Of course, Freud points out that the term "repression" is not relevant in the case of trauma, but when repression takes place, it reveals what is going on unbeknownst to us.

Psychoanalysis, or a recycling sorting system

However, the process takes time. Today, taking time is no longer in style, and techniques of sorting have progressed. Threatened by an impending apocalypse, humanity has learned to sort the trash. Lengthy talking cures are outdated. It's just not possible to return to the time before the French and American Revolutions, when the contents of chamber pots flew out the window, while fears were broached slowly, around the fireplace, in rooms without electricity, through stories about fairies and monsters, in which the knight enters a forest where time stands still.

Today, no one can say, and particularly not in a psychiatric hospital, where and when time stood still. Priorities have been reversed. First, there is sorting for green, black, and yellow garbage bins for recyclable, non-recyclable, and toxic trash. Then, there is psychic sorting carried out at the increasingly rapid rate of diagnoses, prognoses, and illness-specific drugs. The entire matter is settled in ten minutes. The era of analysis of repressed material is over; we are now reprocessing psychic trash: recyclable, non-recyclable, or toxic. A quick pesticide attack and the cockroaches are gone!

As a result, Psyche finds herself, *volens nolens*, accused of impeding sustainable management of the planet, and of polluting the groundwater with all the poisons she spits out. Post-modern man's *hubris* even goes so far as to envisage reducing energy costs by producing genetically modified psyches. But before the gods seek revenge, would it not be advisable to ask ourselves if it is wise to chuck the old cathartic tools that used to help Psyche survive?

Of course, ceremonial traditions are still on display in certain parts of the world, where sometimes native populations are paid to entertain tourists. But what of psychoanalysis? Although tourists in the land of thought still consider it exotic, no one finds it interesting any more. On the contrary. "Sweep it away!" is what we hear everywhere, coming from psychotropic drug trusts, as well as fashionable intellectuals. Will psychoanalysis suffer the same fate as Enlightenment, which today stands accused of consuming too much energy, and whose fatal destiny was predicted by Jonathan Swift before it even came into being?

Man is a broomstick

We have only to refer to his *Meditation upon a Broomstick* (Swift, 1711), which announces the current planetary "spring cleaning". Swift's theorem, "Surely, mortal man is a broomstick!", written in capital letters, indicates that man is a cathartic animal, prone to ridding himself of psychic pollution. Swift's demonstration is based on a carnival ritual of inversion: "But a broom-stick, perhaps you'll say, is an Emblem of a Tree standing on its Head."

The head-to-tail act dear to the theatre of fools revealed, before Freud's time, our repressed desires: "and pray what is Man, but a Topsy-turvy Creature, his Animal Faculties perpetually a Cock-Horse and Rational; His Head where his Heels should be"?

Whether we like it or not, the children's hobby horse, that of May games in Merry England, passed down to Swift's disciple Laurence Sterne (1999), ends up "kindling the flames which warm others".

This sacrificial ritual leads us to reflect on another modern phenomenon. Soon, it will become impossible to throw cigarette ashes on the pavement without some informer catching you in the act of committing the murder inscribed in large letters on the tobacco package. And yet, the ashes of your dear departed can stay on the dresser, the refrigerator, in the closet, or be scattered anywhere, without anyone taking offence. And the bereaved, diagnosed with depression, can purchase the new anti-everything drugs whose sales are skyrocketing in our Western countries.

And since we are constantly told that we have a duty to remember, let us remember Neanderthal man. What does he think of the sad state of the symbolic sphere he worked so hard to clear out, in order to bequeath his burial sites to us? He must be utterly disheartened, beyond the grave, to see his great nephews return to the pre-protohistoric age, even prior to that of mammoths, who were able to impart their burial traditions to elephants! Unless we expect to save the planet with our ashes, scattered to serve as organic fertiliser.

In his *Meditation*, Swift warns us of the risks related to such a thorough house-cleaning: "and yet, with all his faults, [man] sets up to be a universal reformer and corrector of abuses, a remover of grievances, rakes into every slut's corner of nature, bringing hidden corruption to the light, and raises a mighty dust where there was none before; sharing deeply all the while in the very same pollution he pretends to sweep away."

If we keep on overhauling psychic health with a sweep of the broom or a dose of narcotics, we are going to raise the dreaded dust of the unburied dead, who will land in a frenzy on our grandchildren. We are trying to sweep away madness as if it were some kind of pollution, instead of letting it do its cathartic work of resistance to the erasure of traces.

Don Quixote's renewable psychic energy

"Sweep it away!" a forger shouts in Cervantes' ear. The fake sequel to his knight's adventures is not only stupid, but also insulting to him. It calls him old and "one-handed", a reactionary old fossil. Perhaps Cervantes realises that ogres and evil giants exist not only in wars and bagnios, but also in his neighbourhood. He is no doubt wavering on the brink of non-being, which almost engulfed him in his youth. Today, a friend would give him half a pill of this or five grams of that, to prevent him from going berserk. But in the seventeenth century, saving energy was not yet considered useful, so these insults impelled Cervantes to write his own sequel to the adventures, with all due haste.

Forced into a corner, Cervantes has no choice but to call Don Quixote to the rescue. He can't resist sending his knight off on a third sally, propelled out of the cocoon in which he had left him firmly ensconced at the end of the first novel, between his niece, the housekeeper, the barber, and the curate. After all this time, he is a bit worried that he might not recognise his son. But he finds his hero true to his image, although "so withered and dried up that he looked as if he had been turned into a mummy" (De Cervantes, 1605/1615, p. 401). Fortunately, his silhouette has remained unchanged.

Untainted by the chemistry that would have turned him into a wreck, the knight is ready to enter into new transferences. This virginity with respect to medicating drugs was proudly claimed recently in Boston by the author of the best-seller *I Never Promised You a Rose Garden* (1989) by Joanne Greenberg. Treated for schizophrenia after the war, before the medication trend introduced in the 1950s, she was a young girl in the grip of madness when she met Frieda Fromm-Reichmann, herself a survivor of Nazi persecution.

Frieda became acquainted with Quixotic transference in Koenigsberg, Prussia, where she unofficially headed a ward of soldiers with head wounds during the First World War. When she immigrated to the United States in 1937, she was given a summer job at Chestnut Lodge, where she and her friend Harry Stack Sullivan developed the premises of the psychoanalysis of psychosis. It was there that she addressed her famous "I never promised you a rose garden" to Joanne Greenberg, then her young patient, worried about being released after a lengthy hospitalisation. Twenty years later, the story of this analytic adventure became a best-seller translated the world over, except in France.

Cervantes does not promise his son a rose garden either when he sends him off on his third sally. But where can the knight draw his energy from after the mistreatment that left him groggy? This is what we must elucidate to formulate, in our turn, our modest proposal for a solution to the world's energy problems, at least at the psychic level.

Crossing the Lake of Boiling Pitch

The universal success of the first Don Quixote is undoubtedly due to its role in the psychotherapy of war traumas affecting people all over the world, without exception. From the start, in the Author's Preface, Cervantes asserts his intention to combat melancholia by appealing to the god of laughter. At the end of the book, the story of the "Lake of Boiling Pitch" (De Cervantes, 1605/1615, p. 15) describes psychic regeneration in those who stared death in the face.

In the Second Part, Cervantes operates a change in the mission with which he entrusts his son. Of course, the pace is less lively, since both of them are ten years older. They acknowledge the damage wrought by the sly trick neither of them saw coming. Does this mean that the catharsis in the first novel was a failure? Cervantes reviews all of its stages, to identify its weak points.

First, like all soldiers exposed to trauma, the knight plunges into the hell of war, a lake of boiling pitch full of repugnant, foul-smelling creatures. But at the bottom of the lake, there lies a landscape of prairies and gardens surrounding a castle, from which emerge, to greet him, ravishing damsels. "The fairest of them all" not only takes him by the hand, but strips him naked, to wash away his stains. She restores his countenance, but does not promise him "a rose garden" either.

Finally, when he believes he has reached utmost bliss and is "picking his teeth perhaps as usual", a damsel even lovelier than the others appears unexpectedly and asks him to deliver her from a monster. This damsel, bearing a certain kinship with Dulcinea, is not maternal; she urges him to re-enter the social realm through the basic link of the gift.

Cervantes has followed closely the stages of Psyche's psychoanalysis as it is described by Apuleius (1999). When she is left exposed on a rock to be found by a monster, because of Venus's jealousy, Eros falls in love with her and has Zephyr carry her to a castle surrounded by a garden, where she awakens. The god of love, in love with Psyche, brings her back to life. He visits her every night, on condition that she does not try to see him.

Her envious sisters, who wish her dead, convince her to sneak a look at her lover while he sleeps. This scene is depicted in a number of Renaissance paintings. Psyche is awed by the beauty of Eros. As she gazes upon him, a burning drop of oil from the lamp she holds falls on his body and awakens him. Psyche loses her love because she did not keep her promise. Cervantes, like Psyche, did not keep his promise to the last damsel encountered at the bottom of the Lake of Boiling Pitch.

For indeed, this story told in chapter fifty of the first novel is his own story. He too had emerged from a hell full of ghastly creatures, which almost swallowed him up forever. In the last quarter of the book, Cervantes appears at the inn, in the guise of the Captive who has survived the bagnios in Algiers (De Cervantes, 1605/1615, p. 277). There, his son, Don Quixote, is given the place of honour at the kitchen table and, like Aby Warburg, he gives a one-hour lecture entitled "Discourse on Arms and Letters". His audience, made up of gentlemen who follow the profession of arms, listens with great interest and, having heard him, can no longer consider him a madman (De Cervantes, 1605/1615, p. 284).

When Don Quixote, locked in his cage, tells the canon the story of the Lake of Boiling Pitch, he makes it clear that he knows he was snared by the author, his stepfather, since, as he says, "I have seen myself shut up in a cage like a madman" (De Cervantes, 1605/1615, p. 375).

Contributing to the common fate of those diagnosed with mental illness, Cervantes turns away from transference. Worse still, he turns the knight's masked friends against him, and grants amnesty to the rapist Don Fernando, reproducing what often happens in post-war periods.

But Don Quixote, in his madness, knows that the war goes on. This is why, from his cage, he raises a hue and cry to demand that the trappings of knight-errantry be returned to him, so that he might take up the science of chivalry again. Soon Cervantes will come to understand that not only has he betrayed his promise to the hero, but also his promise to a Lady.

The violated letter

In what cage has Cervantes entrapped himself? By locking the knight up, he has imprisoned his own writing in the discourse that holds madness to be incurable. Once crazy, always crazy! No matter what Don Quixote has achieved, how great his courage, how kind his heart, and how remarkable his intelligence, at the end of the novel he is reduced to the stain, the *mancha*, to a psychic defect. Presumably, a psycho-gene will be passed on unchanged for all the centuries to come, amen! Deliver us, Almighty God, from the gene of stupidity!

Like parents tired of their children's antics, Cervantes wants to get away, to travel, leaving his lumbering son at home in the care of a team worthy of institutional approval. Since he has long ago abandoned his plans to immigrate to America, he is now embarked on a Jules Vernian journey between the Mediterranean and Norway, writing his *Persiles* (1914). But it is impossible to sequester the cut-out unconscious. Even though he is now shut away, Don Quixote remains a witness who knows that his father has not freed the last damsel. Who is she?

> The thirteenth returns .... Once more she is the first;
> And she is still the only one, or is this the only moment;
> For you are surely queen, first and last?

... is the question posed by Nerval (1854), the poet abandoned by his mother, who died on the roads of Poland while she followed her husband, a military doctor engaged in Napoleon's campaigns.

We must face facts. Cervantes' work fell into the hands of a forger after it was left defenceless on the open highways of the publishing world. Turned into a Lady without Mercy, the thirteenth damsel reproaches him for his abandonment, and forces Cervantes to defend her anew from the monsters who hide in the calm waters of peacetime. Even now that, as he says himself, he is poor and in ill health, the relentless duena keeps after him.

Let us take stock: the novel has fallen into the hands of barbarians, but what is worse, Dulcinea has been taken hostage and manhandled by a mediocre and vulgar style! For Cervantes, she is not a distant damsel, but literature itself. Thanks to her, he was able to survive the torments of slavery, and to read all the books he could find in Algiers, where they circulated as part of the booty of pirates (Garcés, 2002, p. 66). Upon his return to Spain, she was the inspiration for his plays and for a pastoral romance. And he has let her be violated by a vulgar forger who calls him an old coot!

Cervantes protests: "it is not with grey hairs that one writes, but with the understanding, and that commonly improves with years, [....] I take it amiss, too, that he calls me envious [...], as if I were ignorant [of] what envy is" (2013, p. 397).

This time, the goal is clear. Cervantes will target envious perversion. There is not a moment to lose. He has no time to feel sorry for his son, to ask his forgiveness, or to confess that deep down he loves him just the same. In this family, displays of filial love are not customary. But, by bringing him out of his forced reclusion to impel him to take up arms again, the father admits that his son's madness is the best weapon against perversion.

The challenge of the second part

Cervantes is furious, despite what he says in the Preface, where he displays detachment: "Thou wouldst have me call him ass, fool, and malapert, but I have no such intention."

Although he appears calm, he is on the brink of going berserk, as often happens to soldiers betrayed by their own. Instead of forgiving offences as would befit someone who is, like him, about to enter the Franciscan Order, he takes up the challenge of creating a "Don Quixote continued, and at length dead and buried, so that no one may dare to bring forward any further evidence against him" (De Cervantes, 1605/1615, p. 399).

But the burial will not take place before seventy-four new chapters are written in a style contrasting with our current taste for victimisation. The link between the first novel and the second lies in "having spirit enough to say nay", as it was asserted in the chapter about the convicts: "for, say they, ‹*nay*› has no more letters in it than ‹yea›" (De Cervantes, 1605/1615, p. 137). In the first novel, a "nay" has been opposed to the erasure of the traces of traumas no one wants to hear about. In the Second Part, a "nay" will be proffered, even under torture, to refuse any distortion of these traces.

But first, Cervantes must retrieve his knight from the wastebasket where he tossed the unsatisfactory drafts of a sequel to his book (De Cervantes, 1605/1615, p. 421). When Don Quixote expresses concern about his future fate, the bachelor Sanson Carrasco replies that "no second part has ever been good, and [...] enough has already been written about Don Quixote". And what does the author mean to do?" asks Don Quixote, worried that after having locked him in a cage, the author who brought him into being has lost faith in him. Sanson answers: "Why, as soon as he has found the history which he is now searching for with extraordinary diligence, he will at once give it to the press, moved more by the profit that may accrue to him from doing so than by any thought of praise" (De Cervantes, 1605/1615, p. 421).

And Sancho immediately comments that the author is indeed eager for money. Still, Cervantes would not have written these lines if he had not already found the story he wants to tell.

But what is this profit, greater than any desire for praise? Instead of taking the advice of advertising experts looking to create a publicity stunt, he risks his reputation by confronting an enemy worse than those he faced in war or in slavery, worse than the banker who sent him to the prison of Sevilla: a true editorial trauma inflicted by the literary world where he believed he could seek shelter. This betrayal revives injuries that his age has not erased. Cervantes is not waging the same battle, as he tells us from the start, in the Preface.

Turning to the reader: Cervantes entrusts him with a special mission

Up to this point, Don Quixote, impelled by his hallucinatory visions of events erased from history, rushed ahead first and only later analysed his deeds with Sancho, while they both lay on the ground exhausted. But now anti-personnel landmines are hidden in the discourse heard in reassuring surroundings. The new war on fraud is no longer a direct confrontation.

In the calm before the storm, Cervantes gets ready to fight an invisible enemy. Nothing can deter the elite soldier Cervantes will proudly claim to be until the end of his life. Right from the Preface, the reader is summoned to a briefing where he hears about a battle plan—barely suggested, since the mission is secret—and learns that he is the one recruited to carry it out. Whether we like it or not, we have to take action. Cervantes, the warrior, is ready to provide the necessary training to the new recruits of future centuries (Canavaggio, 2005).

There has been a change of strategy: this time the author involves us in a ruthless battle against the villain, without asking for our consent. When he called us "idle" readers in the Preface to the first novel, we were hardly offended, since he showed himself so modest, with his *captatio benevolentiae*, confessing his anguish in front of the blank page, and his dread of the critics. But now, encouraged by his success, Cervantes no longer minces words. Taken to task right from the start, we are accused of passively awaiting the controversy to come, and then, before we can defend ourselves, we are requested to play a role of go-between, even before reading the book: to tell the forger Cervantes' way of seeing things.

How can we resist responding to Cervantes' impetuous energy, which shakes us out of our chronic depression? As soon as we read the first page, we cannot help being drawn in. Like an old master of the warrior's art—*Budo* in Japanese—Cervantes, despite his age, summons up our vital energy—*ki* in Japanese, *chi* in Chinese—with no apparent effort. In fact, the second novel contains very few of the show-of-force scenes that punctuated the first one. The old knight seems to have calmed down.

This change of pace could be attributed to the fatigue of a man in his sixties. But this is not it at all. As Clausewitz would say, the second novel requires continuing the war through recourse to other means: a martial art learned in the bagnios, which Cervantes leaves it to the knight to teach to us.

After having chosen a name for himself in the first novel, Don Quixote now finds himself "renowned". In chapter III, he will express his surprise to the bachelor Sanson Carrasco, who falls to his knees before him: "So, then, it is true that there is a history of me, and that it was a Moor and a sage who wrote it?" (De Cervantes, 1605/1615, p. 415).

In fact, his lanky silhouette and that of his plump squire are already the highlight of many public celebrations in Spain and abroad. Their story is popular among people of all ages, from the youngest to the oldest: "the children turn its leaves, the young people read it, the grown men understand it, the old folk praise it" (De Cervantes, 1605/1615, p. 418), the bachelor confirms.

But these "foul-mouthed trumpets of glory", as Georges Brassens calls them in one of his songs, are apt to produce the distorted images Cervantes calls false testimony. Thus, just before he died in 1616, at the age of sixty-nine, two years after the publication of the Second Part of *Don Quixote*, Cervantes passed down to his son, *in extremis*, the art of waging psychological war against brainwashing, which we now call "mind control" (Stein, 2010, pp. 251–277).

Escaping the fascination of the mirror

First lesson: whether the reader be "gentle or plebeian", he must not expect to find "retaliation, scolding, and abuse against the author [...] begotten at Tordesillas" (De Cervantes, 1605/1615, p. 397). There is no need for a committee in support of Cervantes. Like a Zen master who castigates visitors unable to get out of dualistic impasses, Cervantes rids us of any desire to take up his cause: "Well then, the truth is, I am not going to give thee satisfaction; for, though injuries stir up anger in humbler breasts, in mine the rule must admit of an exception."

What exactly is this Cervantian exception? First, it helps us understand the intricacies of the perversion to which he was exposed in Algiers, where expressing anger at the offences one suffered led directly to impalement. Still, Cervantes cannot bear the portrayal made of him: "What I cannot help taking amiss is that he charges me with being old and one-handed."

He is proud of his wrinkles and of his hand maimed in battle, that much is clear. But so far we have no idea of the mission with which he entrusts us in regard to the fake author. He barely mentions it: "If perchance thou shouldst come to know him, tell him from me that I do not hold myself aggrieved" (De Cervantes, 1605/1615, pp. 397–398). For the rest, we are left in suspense: "Thou needst say no more to him, nor will I say anything more to thee" (De Cervantes, 1605/1615, p. 399).

But what exactly should we do? Are we to focus on the recurring theme of honour? Don Quixote spoke of nothing else, but now Cervantes appeals to *our* honour. For what purpose? *A word to the wise!* We would like to learn from him what to say to this scoundrel to whom he does not even deign to speak. But no, the elite soldier only reveals his strategy in a veiled manner: "bear in mind that this *Second Part of Don Quixote* which I offer thee is cut by the same craftsman and from the same cloth as the *First*" (De Cervantes, 1605/1615, p. 399).

Like the map in *Treasure Island*, the secret plot of Cervantes is inscribed like a palimpsest in what we read. Recruited against our will, we must shed light on this mystery.

At first glance, it is easy to see in the second novel the use of elements of the first, but the focus is different. For instance: the use of mills (water mills this time), the suicide of a shepherd (but feigned), an encounter with bandits (but Catalan), the braying of asses instead of the bleating of sheep, the return of Gines de Pasamonte as a puppet master, an encounter with Death on the road (but in a play staged by an itinerant theatre), noblemen even more perverse than before, even greener pastoral scenes, duelling that ends badly. This time, the traveller's destination is Catalonia, and specifically the port of Barcelona, where the abduction of the author by Ottoman pirates took place; this event, an abduction not mentioned in the tale of the captive narrated in the first novel, will now be inscribed in black and white. Multiple echoes that nevertheless do not provide the key to the novel we are about to read …

And what about Cervantes' coup in hijacking the reader, driven as he is by his rage to write? Is it the act of a desperate man? Possibly. His work has gotten away from him, Dulcinea is perhaps dreaming of show-business fame. As a result, the four-footed Quixotic transference—involving the knight, Sancho, their mounts, and Dulcinea—is limping. Soon, Sancho's lie will render it even more wobbly. Quite logically, Cervantes leaves it to us to be the spare tyre. In the very first pages, like Baudelaire, he appeals to the "hypocrite reader—my twin—my brother!" (2011), to compel him to speak to this anonymous fellow who does not value the given word.

Even before turning to us, in a fit of rage, Cervantes has rejected several sources of support—and not the least substantial. In his Dedication (p. 395), he confesses to the Count of Lemos that, due to the fame of Don Quixote's adventures, the Emperor of China asked him "to found a college where the Spanish tongue would be taught", and where the book that would be read would be his novel. Although briefly tempted by the offer, Cervantes refused the position of rector at Peking University, indignant that His Majesty had not offered any financial retribution. He was certainly not going to beg for remuneration. He tells the messenger to inform the Emperor that "besides being ill, [he is] very much without money [and that] without so many petty title of colleges and rectorships", he prefers the glory he won at twenty-four, when he was wounded in the

Battle of Lepanto, in October 1571. If the Emperor of China had been ignorant of Quixotic logic, he now knows what to expect.

Entrusted with writing the approbation for the Second Part of Don Quixote, licentiate Marquez Torres confirms Cervantes' statement. In his evaluation, "longer than customary", he recounts how he caused French gentlemen, ardent admirers of Cervantes, to be disillusioned. Having come to Spain with French ambassador Noël Brûlart de Sillery to arrange the marriage between Louis XIII and Anne of Austria, these gentlemen imagined that Cervantes had a subsidy from the Spanish Royal Treasury. "I found myself forced to tell them that he was old, a soldier, a gentleman, and poor" (Canavaggio, 1991, pp. 300–301).

Torres' insistence on the fact that it would have been impossible for Miguel to play the role of a courtesan indicates that he read the Second Part of the novel, in which Cervantes plunges his characters into the troubled waters of a Ducal Court, a place they will have to leave with their heads held high. But how? This is the question that the reader, a reluctant go-between, does not even have the time to ask.

Two stories of fools

Right from the start, in the Preface, Cervantes suddenly makes us step through the looking glass. Two stories of fools are supposed to convey the message to decipher, through offensive madmen who mistreat dogs. Up to this point, we did not dislike Don Quixote's madness, even when it was violent. Has Cervantes redefined the limits of dangerosity, confusing those whom the Argentinian analyst Pichon-Rivière calls *locos lindos*, kind fools, with those he calls *locos di mierda*, vicious knaves? It's hard to believe. Let us try another hypothesis.

To give us some training, Cervantes starts by immersing us in the theatre of fools—called "Sotties" in France—in which the jesters were called by numbers. Fool number 1, and then Fool number 2, burst onto the scene, each of them with a dog and an injunction addressed to us: "I will beg of you [...], to tell him this story" (De Cervantes, 1605/1615, p. 398).

"Him" is the forger to whom we are instructed to tell these two nonsensical stories. Little does it matter if we understand them or not. Has Cervantes become cynical after the hardships he has endured? Possibly, since "cynicism" did not always mean insensitive amorality. On the contrary, according to Antisthenes, Diogenes' master, "For the conduct of life we need right reason or a halter" (1992, p. 67).

In effect, Cervantes' dog stories are in the tradition of the cynic philosophers, whose name is derived from the Athenian gymnasium of Cynosarges, which means "place of the white dog", and above all because "they barked against those in power". Cervantes, who apparently displays Olympian serenity, will in fact bark through the agency of a dog. But we hesitate to form the chorus which joins in. Not that women readers would be excluded from the pack: again according to Antisthenes, the cynics liked intelligent women. So let us shed some light on the situation.

First, we have to become acquainted with the mastery of gestures of the theatre of jesters: the "jest", dear to English readers of Cervantes, Shakespeare, Swift, and Laurence Sterne, takes us back to what Antisthenes called "the action that matters most in speech". But we are struck with stage fright, baffled by the tricks the master pulls out of Diogenes' barrel.

Let us go back to system "phi" in Freud's *Project*. When the word, taken hostage by impostors, loses its value, when the Lady of one's thoughts is about to faint, Psyche is overwhelmed. Cervantes then goes back to the primary process, where words are taken for things, in hopes that they may fall on the ears of the wise. Bion, another war veteran, made similar use of his famous "grid" as a filter through which formulated "alpha" elements are sometimes transformed back into unformulable "beta" elements (Bion, 1983).

Staging "the action that matters most in speech", the two absurd fool stories are intended to create a place of retreat where we can hear Cervantes' silent cries, and deliver him from an enemy. A word to the wise!

In theory, we can easily agree. But when we read the two tales that Cervantes asks us to pass on, we lose all desire to help. As for him, he enjoys telling us what to do. Then, seeing that we are not very amused by the first story, he tries to divert us with an even more provocative one. We have no choice; Cervantes has made his decision. In the unlikely event that we should one day meet the knave of Tordesillas, we will have to tell him the two Andalusian stories that follow.

First story: "there was a madman in Seville …

> … who took to one of the drollest absurdities and vagaries that ever madman in the world gave way to".

Fool number 1's technique is described in detail, in case we find the trick so funny that we want to try it ourselves. The Sevillian "[caught] a dog in the street, […], with his foot held one of its legs fast, and with his hand lifted up the other, and as best he could fixed the tube where, by blowing, he made the dog as round as a ball; then […], he gave it a couple of slaps on the belly, and let it go" (De Cervantes, 1605/1615, p. 398).

A trick not for the faint of heart, in the purest Carnival tradition. Wittgenstein, a faithful reader of Cervantes, would surely ask: What is shown that cannot be said? The speech bubble in the cartoon comes out of the mouth of the fool speaking to the crowd: "Do your worships think, now, that it is an easy thing to blow up a dog?"

What could this mean? Cervantes clarifies the matter in a triumphant tone: "Does your worship think now, that it is an easy thing to write a book?"

And he laughs at his own joke. Your worship, your worship! I, the worship he addresses, conclude after much thought that the novel *Don Quixote* was buggered by a moron whose reputation is overblown by media fanfare. Is our interpretation right? Cervantes does not care and goes on to a second story.

As early as the 1930s, Wittgenstein commented that "psychoanalysis is a very powerful mythology [which requires] very strong and keen and persistent criticism to see through [it]" (1966, p. 41). The philosopher knew very well that traditional analysis did not concur with his experiences as a veteran of the First World War, nor with those of patients in asylums, because: "it is not self-evident to say something to someone" (1953). Wittgenstein was urging analysts to find the paradigm that he was trying to suggest to them: "what cannot be said" can only be shown, using what he calls an "ostensive definition". In 1938, Wittgenstein asked his former student Maurice O'Connor Drury—whom he had advised to become a doctor rather than a philosopher—to arrange for him to visit the psychiatric ward of St Patrick Hospital in Dublin, where long-stay patients were housed. After having spoken with them, Wittgenstein gave Drury this advice: "Always take a seat beside the patient's bed. Don't stand there like the statue of the Commander. Make him feel that he can take the time to talk to you."

In 1946, Wittgenstein stated that "Madness need not be regarded as an illness. Why shouldn't it be seen as a sudden change of character?" (Drury, 1981, p. 121). In fact, this startling change of character occurs when there is no one there with whom to speak. "You say that you have a vague impression, I do not doubt what you say, but I ask you in what game you utter this word? […] In situations where we are tempted to say: I must have gone mad, the old language-game no longer applies" (Wittgenstein, 1934–1936, pp. 275–320).

It is urgent to find a new agreement concerning that which is shown because it cannot be said. But what agreement does Cervantes seek when he insists on another ostensive definition, in another story of madness, even more shocking than the first? Like Diogenes, he is not concerned with pleasing us, and even less with soliciting compassion.

Second story: "in Cordoba, there once was another madman, ...

> ... whose way it was to carry a piece of marble slab or a stone, not of the lightest, on his head".
>
> (De Cervantes, 1605/1615, p. 398)

The madman of Cordoba is much more alarming than his Sevillian counterpart. He crushes "any unwary dog" in sight. This raises terrible howling, which leaves him indifferent, since he does the same thing to the next dog, until he meets up with the behavioural therapy administered by a hot-headed draper, the owner of a lurcher.

The technique consists of a memorable beating punctuated by the word "lurcher": "snatching up a measuring yard [he] rushed out at the madman and [...] at every stroke he gave him he said, 'You dog, you thief! My lurcher! Don't you see, you brute, that my dog is a lurcher?'" (De Cervantes, 1605/1615, p. 398).

A foreshadowing of our modern miraculous short-term therapies! Which work! Well, perhaps not so well, since the madman "came out again with his old trick and a heavier load than ever. He came up to where there was a dog, and [examined] it very carefully." Since the word "lurcher" was associated with the beating he received, the madman held himself back from dropping the stone, no matter what sort of dog he saw, because "all the dogs he came across, be they mastiffs or terriers, he said were lurchers". But what exactly is Cervantes getting at?

Eureka! Once again, the dog represents the abused novel. Treated like carrion, blown up, deformed, crushed, the book was released into the world howling with pain. Cervantes aches for his violated novel and threatens to take revenge. "Maybe it will be the same with this historian, that he will not venture another time to discharge the weight of his wit in books, which, being bad, are harder than stones" (De Cervantes, 1605/1615, p. 398).

Little does it matter now whether the two madmen are offensive or not. By telling these stories, Cervantes introduces the ferocity of the theatre of fools, to proclaim that "the poor man may retain honor, but not the vicious" (De Cervantes, 1605/1615, p. 399).

Honour is restored to a mind that few can equal, even if they have become masters in the art of buggering and crushing. Whether they come from literary circles—to which the forger is said to belong—or from the bagnios of Algiers, those who force Dulcinea into prostitution deserve nothing but cudgel blows. Cervantes conveys this to the reader, in his veiled style: "for I know well what the temptations of the devil are, and that one of the greatest is putting into a man's head that he can write and print a book by which he will get as much fame as money, and as much money as fame" (De Cervantes, 1605/1615, p. 398).

If he would have raised a furious hue and cry about the theft and violation of his book, Cervantes would have received the same diagnosis that was given to his son. This is why he advises the reader: "Thou needst say no more to him."

Once these two condensed scenes are enacted, we are told nothing more. But when the curtain rises on the opening scene of the novel, we know that Cervantes has drafted us, like he drafted his son, into a political arena. After dissuading us from responding to an attack by imitating the strategy of the aggressor, Cervantes now shows us how to escape the ministrations of those who want to pacify us.

Don Quixote's discharge: the psychiatric exam

First, the patient must be released after hospitalisation at the request of a third party. This is no easy task. In chapter I, when we entered the hero's house, we penetrated into a domain where there is no more hope, for the treatment of the madman stops time, instituting "chronicity". Don Quixote, who already lived in a time dimension of his own, is now forced to live in a monotony intended to stop delusions. "I am an old chronic psychotic", used to tell me a beautiful forty-year-old woman, raped in adolescence and continuously discouraged from uncovering her story, which counted for so little in the eyes of modern versions of Doctor Thomas Diafoirus.

Cervantes starts by making a distinction between Don Quixote's out-of-time and out-of-place exploits, and the out-of-history immobility forced upon him by his team of caregivers. God save the team! When the barber and the curate visit him for the mandatory follow-up exam after the first month of confinement, they are careful to erase his history with a piece of judicious medical advice. "they agreed not to touch upon any point [that should] bring back to his recollection what had taken place" (De Cervantes, 1605/1615, p. 399).

To avoid excitement, their patient must not know what is happening outside either. Considered a mentally ill patient no longer in crisis, his only horizon is stupour. In fact, his caregivers are careful to avoid informing him of the success of his adventures, for fear of exciting him. A proper psychiatric examination is carried out by these learned gentlemen. Since the patient "[was] beginning to show signs of being in his right mind [...] they resolved to pay him a visit and test the improvement in his condition, although they thought it almost impossible that there could be any". Today, certificates signed after a month of hospitalisation often express the same reservations.

The examiners' caution allows Don Quixote to pass the clinical exam with flying colours. Standing behind their one-way mirror, the surgeons of the soul observe the scars left by the trauma after confinement, and "this gave [them] great satisfaction [...] and they agreed not to touch upon any point connected with knight-errantry so as not to run the risk of reopening wounds which were still so tender". Their theory, already then, was that delusional states are due to brain lesions and are subordinated to a magic formula such as: madness drives a man mad as surely as rope hangs the hanged man. Therefore, one must not speak to a madman of his madness any more than one should speak of a rope in the house of a hanged man.

Mum's the word, then, especially regarding what's most important. The two healers of the body and soul speak to their patient about this and that, that is to say, about politics. "so completely did they remodel the State, that they seemed to have thrust it into a furnace and taken out something quite different from what they had put in". Like patrons of a pub putting the world to rights, they corrected or condemned abuses of various kinds, "reforming one practice and abolishing another [...]; and on all the subjects they dealt with, Don Quixote spoke with such good sense that the pair of examiners were fully convinced that he was quite recovered and in his full senses" (De Cervantes, 1605/1615, p. 401).

Believing firmly, before their time, in a scientific paradigm, they do not see that things are about to change. Happily for us, and for the good of the Republic, Don Quixote's red and green garb alerts us that madness is about to enter the scene, despite its mummification. How will Cervantes proceed in order to draw his son out of the chronicity in which so many talented old children are stuck?

He will raise the question of a cure for madness, a possibility still regarded with great scepticism. "changing his original plan, the curate resolved to test Don Quixote's recovery thoroughly, and see whether it was genuine or not". The experiment was just as banal then as it is now, for everyone already knew how to trigger post-traumatic stress disorder.

The curate suggests, innocently, that "the Turk was coming down with a powerful fleet", a fact that would continue to be true for several more centuries on Mediterranean shores. Just what was needed to produce the desired effect? "Do you want me to wind him up?" used to ask a nurse in the first asylum where I trained as a psychoanalyst. The madman would then perform his act, with the bored look of an old lion in a circus.

The patient Quixote falls into the trap, like everyone else, aware like they all are of the subterfuge. But he knows that his battle is no longer to be fought with drawn sword, and he is careful not to say too much. "[My advice], master shaver, will not be impertinent, but, on the contrary, pertinent."

But he refuses to reveal his advice. Irked by his resistance, the two inquisitors subject him to their battery of tests, assuring him that confidentiality will be respected. "'My profession,' replied the curate, '[…] is to keep secrets'" (De Cervantes, 1605/1615, p. 403).

Today, the same specialists identify in nursery schools the agitated tots who must be given drugs to keep the markets moving, while granting parents confidentiality. This double-dealing has become so common that no one takes notice any more. The only ones who rebel are those whose traumas have rendered them hypervigilant, and who, like Don Quixote, are impelled to voice a rallying cry: "all the knights-errant that are scattered over Spain [should be commended] to assemble in the capital, for […] there may be one among them who alone will suffice to destroy the entire might of the Turk" (De Cervantes, 1605/1615, p. 398).

In the battle against the deceitful experimental game which equates the psyche with a broken machine, the number of warriors is not what counts. Today, the objectivation theory reigns supreme. But Cervantes was already making it clear that the barber and the curate are ignoring transference in their allegedly objective psychiatric assessment.

Thus, the diagnosis of madness is confirmed when Don Quixote, carried away, shows himself ready to deliver the battle single-handedly. Although he does not claim to be as valiant as knights-errant of yore, he is determined not to be inferior in spirit. He is willing to take on the mission his father entrusted to him a few pages back: "God knows what I mean, and I say no more" (De Cervantes, 1605/1615, p. 403).

God knows, as we do, that objectifying madness is the evil Cervantes has chosen to combat. The theory that "it is in the brains" (De Cervantes, 1605/1615, p. 435) continues to be taught today in the most prestigious universities. Nothing much has changed since the courses taught at the University of Salamanca, which, according to Sanson Carrasco, turned out the best graduates. This new character—the student—in the second novel adds credence to the scientistic dogma of the barber and the curate. To illustrate it and discredit it at the same time, Cervantes presents another story of fools narrated by the barber.

Third story of fools: "in the madhouse at Seville ...

> ... there was a graduate in canon law whom his relations had placed there".

After a few years, he felt he had recovered and wanted to be released, especially since he became aware that his relatives were taking advantage of his madness to enjoy his property. The barber tells Don Quixote this story to incite him to resignation. For "this graduate [...] took it into his head that he was sane [...], and under this impression" (De Cervantes, 1605/1615, p. 403), if he thought one can recover from madness, he would soon have to change his mind, and his fate would quickly be sealed.

And yet, the young man is convinced that he is cured. Of course, no one believes him. So he writes a letter to the Archbishop entreating him to have him released from forced confinement. The prelate, "moved by repeated, sensible, well-written letters", directed an expert, "one of his chaplains, to make inquiry of the madhouse as to the truth of the licentiate's statements, and to have an interview with the madman himself" (De Cervantes, 1605/1615, p. 403).

At first, the word of the patient seems to count. Central to the enquiry is the interview, in other words, the transference. The judge in charge of the medical decision, just like Homer's *histor*, "the judge of the judges", could have attested to the reasonableness of the student's request. But, unable to decipher a language game too subtle for him, he diagnoses the student as having a psychotic structure, as Gödel, Cantor, Nash, and other *beautiful minds* (Nasar, 1998) were labelled, including Wittgenstein, if we believe Lacan's remark on the philosopher's "psychotic ferocity" (Lacan, 2001f).

The director of the madhouse naturally expresses doubt about the patient's recovery, for he needs to fill his hospital beds, which were nothing more in Cervantes' time than bunks or cages in wards for turbulent patients. As for his family, his relations were "covetous and heartless", and interested in keeping him where he was. "In order to enjoy [...] his large property, his enemies disparaged and threw doubts upon the mercy our Lord had shown him in turning him from a brute beast into a man", and bribed the governor of the asylum to diagnose him "still mad but with lucid intervals" (De Cervantes, 1605/1615, p. 403).

The student does not mince words when he describes the beast-like condition to which he has been reduced. Today's more polished vocabulary would designate him as a health-care user or even a citizen, but the denigration of his madness remains the same. Like Don Quixote, he passes the first test successfully. The chaplain was convinced, by seeing that "he spoke so rationally", and decided "to take him away with him that the Archbishop might see him, and ascertain for himself the truth of the matter". Indeed, the touchstone of truth is the *leitmotiv* of the two novels.

At first, positive transference develops on the part of the expert. Obeying the order of the Archbishop, he has "the clothes in which the licentiate had entered the house given to him", restoring him to human appearance. At this point, the ordeal of Tantalus begins. Believing he can trust a *therapon* worthy of the name, the young man is confident his torment is over. But the prospect of freedom fades when a sudden change of paradigm transforms this dynamic episode into a definitive diagnosis.

The patient has made a fatal error. As naïve as Don Quixote who believed he could deliver Andrés from his cruel master's whip, the licentiate succumbs to a humanitarian impulse, overlooking the carceral setting. In such a setting, reactions are extreme. "He, as soon as he saw himself [...] divested of the appearance of a madman, entreated the chaplain to permit him in charity to go and take leave of his comrades the madmen" (De Cervantes, 1605/1615, p. 404).

Cervantes must have had the same desire when he thought his liberation was at hand. The chaplain seized upon this opportunity to visit these circles of hell which, for several centuries to come, continued to attract the curious as well as thrill-seekers, until television provided us with a guided tour, sparing us the need to leave our homes. Here, we are taken into the quarters of the raving mad, also described by Swift a century later in his "Digression on madness" (1704).

Psychotic transference

Acting as a therapist, the young man gives hope to his companions in captivity, for he "has gone through it". Proximity and expectancy are two of the four principles defined by Salmon in 1917 for the psychotherapy of trauma. "Have strong hope and trust [in God]. [...] I will take care to send you some good things to eat. [...] Take courage!"

But in this place of hopeless confinement, his benevolent words trigger the envious rage of a lunatic who, hearing this sympathetic farewell: "It is I, brother, who am going [home]", rose from an old mat "on which he lay stark naked" and invoked the evil spirit which reigned in that place: "Mind what you are saying, licentiate; don't let the devil deceive you."

The generosity of the one who can leave can only be rejected by the one who has to stay: "You, cured! well, we shall see; [...] Dost thou not know [...] that I [am], as I say, Jupiter the Thunderer, who hold in my hands the fiery bolts with which I am able and am wont to threaten and lay waste the world?" (De Cervantes, 1605/1615, p. 404).

This is how Ovid describes personified Envy in *The Metamorphoses*: "She finds men's successes disagreeable, and pines away at the sight. She gnaws and being gnawed is also her own punishment" (AD 8, Book II, v. 780). The lunatic rants on, asserting that it will not rain in Seville, "nor on any part of its district or territory, for three whole years [...]. Thou free, thou cured, thou in thy senses! And I mad, I disordered, I bound!" (De Cervantes, 1605/1615, p. 405).

His long stay among madmen has taught the student to play tit-for-tat. In his turn, he becomes Neptune, who can "rain as often as it pleases [him] and may be needful". But this is where he falls into a trap. Fooled by the unctuous demeanour of his saviour, he turns to the chaplain and takes his hands to entrust him with his interpretation: "Be not uneasy, señor; attach no importance to what this madman has said; for if he is Jupiter and will not send rain, I, who am Neptune ..." (De Cervantes, 1605/1615, p. 405).

Despite all his learning and culture, the chaplain is unable to grasp the specificity of transference in psychosis, where mythological poetry resonates. Here, the "subject who is supposed to know", as Lacan (1975) designates the analyst in classical transference, is not relevant.

Since then, Benedetti has made it clear that in order to change the course of madness "one must enter the delusion" (1998) and deflect its deadly effect through a positive transformation. But when the licentiate used this analytic strategy on the threshold of his prison, he did not expect his supervisor to remain rooted in neutrality. The chaplain is far from playing Sancho Panza's therapeutic role. He sentences the recovering patient to life-long confinement, making sarcastic use of the vocabulary of his delusion: "For all that, Senor Neptune, it will not do to vex Senor Jupiter; remain where you are, and some other day, when there is [...] more time, we will come back for you" (De Cervantes, 1605/1615, p. 405).

The verdict was met with great mirth: "The governor and the bystanders laughed, and at their laughter the chaplain was half ashamed" (De Cervantes, 1605/1615, p. 405).

The inflection of a voice was enough to transform positive transference into psychic torture. A word to the wise! The barber insinuates that this is the fate awaiting Don Quixote if he insists on regaining his freedom. "So they stripped the licentiate, and he was left where he was; and that's the end of the story" (De Cervantes, 1605/1615, p. 405).

"La depravada edad nuestra": psychological war

The knight had no trouble recognising the barber's sadistic hint, since he has been well informed by his father, Cervantes, about the tricks played on the slaves in the bagnios. "So that's the story, master barber, [...] which [...] you could not help telling? Master shaver, master shaver! How blind is he who cannot see through a sieve?" (De Cervantes, 1605/1615, p. 405).

Here, the sieve is that of double language, used to intimidate Don Quixote and indirectly dissuade him from undertaking a third sally. But when he made his first two sallies, the knight did not ask anyone's permission. The second book is cut from the same cloth as the first, but now, instead of simply taking off at dawn, Don Quixote must extricate himself from the therapeutic control exercised by his friends.

First, he must free himself from dualism. Here again, Don Quixote is heeding the advice his father offered in the Preface: to escape the fascination of mirrors. He asks the barber: "Is it possible that you do not know that comparisons of wit to wit, valor with valor, beauty with beauty, birth with birth, are always odious and unwelcome?" Like a talisman, this injunction protects against submission, thwarting the "either/or" of closed multiple-choice questioning—wise or foolish?—it opens the field of expectancy: "I, master barber, am not Neptune, the god of the waters, nor do I try to make anyone take me for an astute man, for I am not one" (De Cervantes, 1605/1615, p. 405).

Thus, Don Quixote passes the test of binary labelling with flying colours, and is free to follow his own inclinations. His pupil, Wittgenstein, perpetuates the lesson:

> At the end of my lecture on ethics I spoke in the first person: I think that this is something very essential. Here there is nothing to be stated anymore; all I can do is step forth as an individual and speak in the first person. And here it is essential that this is not a description of sociology but that I am speaking about myself.
>
> (Wittgenstein, 1929)

Don Quixote does not intend to prove or disprove his madness, nor to use it as a Foucaultian argument for liberating the mad; rather, his goal is to combat the perversity of our century: *la depravada edad nuestra*, our depraved age (De Cervantes, 1605/1615, p. 405), in which there is great need for "the protection of damsels, the succour of orphans and minors". Although it appears outdated, this ethical question is, in fact, timely today. When addressing the barber and the curate who reduce him to a medical case, Don Quixote, like Wittgenstein, speaks in the first person. "My only endeavor is to convince the world of the mistake it makes in not reviving in itself the happy time when the order of knight-errantry was in the field."

This well-worn phrase springs to life in the episode where Don Quixote embarks on a journey that today's barbers and curates would call "pathological". For his future adventure, he imagines "a small boat without oars", which will, in fact, appear in chapter XXIX. It will carry him and Sancho to the real castle of the duke and duchess, an illustration of a society of pretence, whose values he deplores: "But now sloth triumphs over energy, indolence over exertion, vice over virtue, arrogance over courage, and theory over practice in arms, which flourished and shone only in the golden ages and in knights-errant" (De Cervantes, 1605/1615, p. 406).

Cervantes entreats us to act as witnesses to the decadence which is growing despite the Golden Age, and against which his son stands up at once. To arms! May God protect him from his friends; as for his enemies, he will take care of them: "And so I will stay where I am, as the chaplain does not take me away."

Without looking for help from any saviour, Don Quixote takes up the dialogue started by the licentiate in the story, precisely at the point where the expert betrayed him. Identifying with Neptune, as the student did, he gives his caregivers a lesson in the use of transference when dealing with madness: "and if Jupiter, as the barber has told you, will not send rain, here am I, and I will rain when I please. I say this that Master Basin may know that I understand him" (De Cervantes, 1605/1615, p. 406). A word to the wise!

Look out! The psychological war has started, waged with kid gloves for the moment, for the time it takes Don Quixote to gather substantial provisions, for body and soul, to sustain him in the battles he has to fight.

Another law student was going to face the same situation five centuries later.

CHAPTER TWO

Bion—Quixote

Time regained: a race against the clock

The analyst had no idea of the battles he would have to fight when the young man with the pale gaze first appeared, as if from nowhere.

It even seemed that he had stepped out of time long ago, since he regularly arrived when he had no scheduled appointment, several hours before the set time, or several hours later; several days before, or several days after. Once, the analyst had thought it well advised to point out that he had come on the right day, at the right hour, seeing this as progress in their relationship, which had been going on for several months. But he answered candidly: "What I think is that I am a week early, or a week late."

Much later, the analyst received the various psychiatric reports that had accompanied his patient's childhood and adolescence. They testified to the stupid alliance between doctors and teachers determined to marginalise him, while acknowledging his surprising intelligence. Especially since his parents could afford to pay for all kinds of private institutions, in addition to what the public school system could offer.

The portrait painted by these reports of different stages in his development is frightening:

> Age eight: motor deficiency with awkwardness and slowness, disorganised writing with stiffness. In addition, orientation and spatial sense problems, as well as emotional inhibition.
>
> Age fifteen: may suffer from inferiority complex. Request for medical opinion concerning general lack of activity. Specific concerns: learning and development difficulties affecting scholastic results.
>
> Age sixteen: development problems and subsequent character instability. Agitation and irritation culminating in need for a period of leave. Recommended that he be sent home for eight days, in hopes that upon his return he will have calmed down and be ready to behave appropriately.
>
> Age seventeen: rehabilitated dyslexic student who changed school five times (in fact, twelve times). Repeated his first year of secondary school, refuses to work. Difficult to conduct psychological evaluation, refuses to cooperate. Intelligence test: superior intelligence, particularly in logic, mathematics and abstract reasoning, where his marks are well above average. Well-read and knowledgeable. Personality: inhibition of emotional life (refuses colours), deficient sense of reality, sexual ambivalence. This deep passivity is cause for concern.

Despite this chaotic scholastic career, he obtained a legal certification, sometimes granted without a secondary study diploma. Since then, he worked as a volunteer at "legal clinics" destined for people who need a lawyer but cannot pay legal fees. This honest young man had even acquired a kind of specialisation in conflicts between landlords and tenants.

He himself lived in a small room in a rather rundown building, in a working-class neighbourhood that had not yet undergone gentrification.

The analyst had trouble identifying his status in society, despite, or due to, the honesty and simplicity of their exchanges. In fact, after a while, he stopped trying; the young lawyer described his meetings with his "patients"—the word was suggested by the analyst—with clinical precision and a sense of humour that kept the demands of the plaintiffs at a certain distance. He always gave them sound advice which sometimes allowed them to avoid risky litigation.

Otherwise, he remained a mystery. Not only was he never on time for his appointments, but he had a great talent for changing his appearance, so that the analyst would often be surprised to find a perfect stranger in the waiting room: new haircut, sometimes a different hair colour, different style of clothing, and, above all, a disposition which seemed adapted to changing circumstances. "The colour of the weather", like that of the dresses of the abused princess in the *Magic Donkey*, if we can invoke such a model to describe this grown-up child, both naïve and remarkably intelligent, who had chosen to step out of our time dimension.

And where was he going now, taking the analyst along—a passenger a bit confused but not worried, who had been able to trust him from the start?

Time was passing, but seemed to stand still. Always the same meetings (in a manner of speaking), not noted in any appointment book; the same pleasant sessions between two people who recognised each other. This pre-existing moment of recognition had probably been needed for time to set itself in motion and take the first step in an ongoing process on which he had to embark with the analyst.

The story of a scale

One day (a red-letter day, as it would turn out), he arrived more unsettled than usual to take his place in the unpredictable space of time of the sessions. The daze of daily life (*L'Écume des jours*, referred to in English as *The Foam of the Daze*, a Boris Vian novel) in his building had just been disturbed by an incident. Several rooms opening onto the same corridor seemed to have been visited, probably by thieves.

But he had not had a chance to speak with his neighbours, drop-outs like him, who had escaped the "perverse occupations" to which "men run panting" as Théophile Gautier writes in his poem "The First Smile of Spring" (1852). We had learned it by heart in nursery school, without knowing that an earlier collection of Gautier's poems, published in 1838, bore the title *The Comedy of Death*. No doubt the analyst could have sensed sooner, behind this smiling innocence, the brush with a faceless death, not cruel but just present enough to prevent the young man from living.

For the moment, the young man seemed distressed. It was easy to guess that his modest refuge was not a model of neatness. He had never "tidied up", and it was easy to imagine that piles of papers and undated letters were strewn everywhere, barely leaving room for the bed. What distressed him most was that nothing seemed to have been taken: the thief must have come off badly in all that mess. Ah, yes, he added, as if in passing, there was, in fact, something that disappeared. It was a whimsical object so far removed from the usual inventory of everyday life that he had trouble identifying it by its name for the analyst. Finally, from his description the analyst concluded that he was speaking of an assay balance. A small pharmacist's or jeweller's scale with a glass cover, for precise measurement, which had landed in his room God knows when or how. In any case, now it was no longer in the junk pile of his familiar things, and its absence created a sort of void. Still, there was no great loss: he had never had occasion to use it and didn't see what use he might possibly have for it in the future.

But the following week his countenance had changed. The analyst was to see this particular expression on his face only twice in the course of their work together. He wore a new mask—as he did when he changed his identity unexpectedly—which bore the imprint of unfathomable fear. Again, he spoke of the scale. He had found it. Did this mean that everything was back in place in this frozen-time world of his? Not at all, for he had visited the room next to his, whose door had been left ajar. This room had been vacant for several months, and he had risked taking a look inside. That's when he saw, out in the open on a table, the assay balance that had vanished. The analyst imagined various detective-novel scenarios that could explain the mystery. The bungling thief could have stolen the scale in question from the young man's room and then left it in the next room, thinking that taking this fragile, bothersome object was not worth the money it would bring.

Still, the young man's gaze remained sombre. One could read in his eyes the most intense fear. His own explanation was more frightening than the analyst's; he supposed that he had moved the scale himself from one room to another. The scale now filled up all the space, including the space of the session, since he did not have the least recollection of having done this. This uncanny event now provided possible confirmation of all the diagnoses of his youth, when experts warned his parents to expect delusions and the personality disturbances indicative of schizophrenia.

At that point, the analyst thought it judicious to say: "Well, this scale wanted to find its way here and take up all this space between us. Perhaps you have made the enormous effort of taking the first step from a place where nothing has budged for a long time. Your story and your fear allow me to give it refuge here, and we shall see what this little scale has to tell us."

In truth, despite saying this, the analyst did not know what to think.

The time swindlers

When thought stops, paralysed by the day-to-day manoeuvres of normality, events start to think in the place of the petrified thinkers. Wilfred Bion described the unfolding of these "thoughts without a thinker".

Between us, these thoughts without a thinker had taken the form of an assay balance. In these strange situations, objects become active participants, like the "objective chance" of the Surrealists (as if chance could also have subjective bearing). They start to revolve around a blind centre—but not as blind as those who will not see.

In the course of that week, the analyst visited some monuments with friends from abroad. In addition, he received a postcard from a colleague on vacation at the other end of the country, bringing the analyst's gaze back to the scale again. Now, it no longer floated in the air, but was held in the hand of a blindfolded allegorical feminine figure. Obviously, the most traditional attributes of Justice were manifest here. Perhaps the scale also suggested the profession of the young patient who lacked patience, since in order to have patience one must dwell in the dimension of time. But he did not have time. He did not have it in his hands, or in his head, or anywhere else.

The analyst hastened to inform him of the majestic arrival of Justice in the field of their work, with the scale held firmly in her hand. The young man did not seem surprised by this discourse that resembled a first attempt to assess the situation—despite its nebulous character—and provide some initial bearing. But from then on, he let it appear clearly that he was starting to settle into a dimension that was new for him, and new for the analyst as well in the context of their relation, based to that point solely on trust—blind trust?—which was mutual.

We were nearing the time of the year when tax returns have to be filed. He was the one who brought up the subject, which was surprising for someone with no revenue other than a meagre allowance from his family. But now, the scale had decided to show, doggedly, a veritable tampering with time.

The analyst was by no means a tax expert, but the deception would have been clear to anyone. Each year, for quite a long while, a transfer of shares made the young man the central depository of the major portion of his father's fortune. Of course, he could in no way benefit from these transactions—"Sign here!"—and as soon as the tax filing period was over, he found himself destitute again, and not even aware that "he" had been rich for a few weeks. Naturally, all this served to avoid paying very high taxes, perhaps without breaking the law, if one is skilled at taking advantage of certain fiscal loopholes. He had only to hand over his identity and his signature for a while, and to continue to shut his eyes and his mouth. All this took place in the open, as he knew, and neither cost him anything nor gave him anything. He had only to do this and, presto!—the law was circumvented with ease, with the murky ease of the "business world". Nothing could be more commonplace. Everyone does it, everyone knows it, Bion would have said, sounding a warning about actual transference.

Of course, it was not the analyst's job to do the work of a tax agent. But, the past few weeks had truly brought the patient and the therapist together. Time is money, they say in the financial world. There are also time-limited investments. But here, the young man had to be given back his time, time stolen, hidden, and abolished by a real manipulation which had turned him into someone who could not say "I".

Thus, the analyst contented himself with forbidding him to participate in this annual scheme, arguing that he could not at once be himself here and appear on a piece of paper as some other person without substance, forced to play the role of nominee in a fiscal swindle. This was their first pact: it went into effect as soon as the analyst stated this injunction in clear terms.

Like storks or swallows, time returns

Starting with his next appointment—and for all the ones that followed—he arrived on time, and on the right day. If he could not make it, he called the analyst in advance. And since he had a sense of humour, as time went on, he displayed on his arm, which had probably never worn watch bands—his personal declaration of freedom—about twenty Swiss plastic watches, some of them enormous and clearly worn to be seen. Neither he nor his analyst ever mentioned them, nor did they ever mention his newfound punctuality.

At about the same time, one of his most loyal friends, who had been his pal through schoolboy days, private tutoring, and law school, offered to hire him to work in a municipal law office whose mission was the same as that which he carried out by providing free legal consultation. He accepted the offer, thus acquiring his first paid job.

No more was heard about the tax-evasion scheme; evidently, a quick solution had been found to his desertion, which must have been interpreted as one more eccentricity on the part of a person experts had always considered disturbed.

But not long afterwards his mother became seriously ill.

Sylvie, five and a half

They had not talked much about his mother until then. But her illness and increasingly alarming relapses led the analyst to try to shed some light on the disquieting mystery surrounding this side of the young man's family. He was able to transmit the analyst's questions directly to his mother during his frequent visits to the hospital, or in the course of her recovery periods. It appeared that she was the only survivor of many children, her brothers and sisters, who had died at an early age. She had vague memories of some of them; as far as the others were concerned, she no longer remembered when or where, or even if, they had been buried. In any case, she liked these conversations with her son, which broke the official silence she had imposed on herself.

But the analyst was alerted by certain details that the transferential process had again become entrapped in some folds of time left unexplored, subjected to non-existence or at least to indifference. On his mother's side, the inheritances were simplified, but these simplifications demanded a price. The young man was part of the price to pay.

Little by little, the sessions, which had nevertheless been enriched by these discussions, seemed to navigate towards an unfathomable past. Even visits to old cemeteries did not provide rekindled energy. Had we no choice but to wait for "the child and the spells" (Ravel, 1925) to make objects speak, sing, and dance, so that the mother's "Be good!" might solicit true emotion that stands a chance of being mutual?

Having learned from previous experience, one day the analyst asked the patient straight off to choose an object present in his everyday life and bring it with him to the session, without waiting for enchanters to move it about. A few days later, this little object appeared in the analyst's office in all its fragility.

All this was taking place at the now far-off time when disposable lighters were starting to enter into unfair competition with matches. As a result, Seita, the match manufacturer, was attempting to build customer loyalty by transforming its little match boxes into collectors' items. One year, the boxes bore children's drawings on their covers: it was one of these that landed in the analyst's office.

The colourful, naive drawing of a small child had been made using awkward but firm lines. Foolishly, the analyst slid the little matchbox open: what was he hoping to find? Of course, the box was empty, and the young man gazed at the analyst with a smile. At least, what the analyst remembered about long-ago deaths in the family gave a certain resonance to the name and age of the young artist: "Sylvie, five and a half". So, it was a little girl named Sylvie who had drawn this portrait reproduced thousands of times, and she had been five and a half when she drew this small child. Was it a self-portrait? Was it the drawing of a new baby in the family? Hopefully, she and her family had benefited from copyrights.

When an analyst does not know what to say, when he foolishly opens an empty box, he starts to listen to the resonance of signifiers. Resonating against the background of the series of deceased children in the maternal line, he could hear "Sylvie", in French, as "*s'il vit*" (if he lives), so that the inscription on the matchbox became "If he lives to five and a half". A pessimistic paediatrician might have predicted that the child would not reach five and a half. Or, on the contrary, the good fairy bending over the cradle may have said that if he survived to that age, he would go on to live a long life.

Faced with the empty box, the analyst was in fact grappling with the fate of children attempting to inscribe themselves in time and who, on occasion, succeed. Simply put, this is called living and, before that, coming into the world. The conclusion reached by the analyst demanded that he take bold steps: he had to explain that having time also meant using one's creative potential. In short, this young man who had lived in almost monastic solitude, but could be at ease in all kinds of social situations, had reached the point in his life where he could hope to create a new time; in other words, he was on the verge of continuing his lineage. The analyst chose to tell him this.

Nothing is easy

But time does what it wants when one tries to go back to its fractures. At first, between the patient and the analyst there had been the compact presence of time that stood still, and sometimes even flowed backwards, adding confusion to immobility. Yet it was not so simple. The analyst was not particularly proud of what was taking place now that a new rhythm had been established, and one could almost see and touch time that had set itself in motion again. Little by little. After he started his new job, the young man moved out of this boundless residence which had sheltered the confusion of time periods and of generations.

Finally, he met a young woman with whom he started a relationship that seemed very fulfilling for both of them.

So, time advanced slowly, like the second hand of the analyst's watch. Moreover, they had settled into a rhythm that revealed a somewhat obsessional manner of doing things. In fact, they were slowly advancing together towards a potential outcome they could not yet describe. For they had not yet really reached the moment when time had come to a standstill, when the past-present did not open onto any future.

The truth is that, little by little, the analyst could not listen to him any more because his head—or rather his ears—had been taken over by a voice that kept saying: "When all is said and done, this man must have a child!" The young man had never spoken about having children, or of not wanting to have children; nor had he said whether he had ever discussed the subject with the woman who shared his life. The analyst started to find the sessions unbearable, because of this obsessive idea that thundered in his ears. Would it not be wise to find some quick way of ending their meetings?

Must the analyst continue to act like an analyst, as sharp-witted patients like to say, meaning continue to say nothing, to indicate to the patient that he can go on talking even though the analyst does not hear him? One day, he finally decided to speak to this reasonable man about the transferential situation in which he found himself: he would simply describe what he was experiencing. As soon as the session began, the analyst announced: "Listen, for some time now I can no longer hear what you are telling me. I can't remember anything you said over the past few weeks because I don't hear you. When you are with me, I can only hear what I have in my head, a strange idea that you never talked to me about: the idea that you should have a child."

Someone else might have gotten up angrily, telling the analyst that he was not there to put up with his projective fancies. But the young man only gazed at him, not even surprised, as if he could hear at that moment what the analyst had to say, and could even identify the strange voice that was speaking these words. He acknowledged softly that this concerned him. Right away, the analyst was able to hear again what the patient was saying, and to remember it easily. This mechanism appeared to have created between them a necessary potential place, and to have voiced words almost impossible to conceive until now, addressed to the young man's companion.

Gods and dogs

After this, the analyst and the young man entered together into another time that resembled waiting. A few months later, when there was still no sign of a pregnancy, he and his companion consulted a gynaecologist and were told not to worry and to give themselves some more time before taking medical measures. "Come back and see me in six months if nothing happens, but I am sure this young lady will be pregnant before long, etc." It was clear that the gynaecologist had not been forced to be in the place of the analyst for months and months. When six months had passed, there was another visit to the doctor and other tests; this time, medical treatment was prescribed, first to the young woman and then to him, based on reasoning the analyst found more and more baffling.

Over a year had passed since the idea of a child had burst on the scene. The analyst was starting to lose patience when the young man recounted his visits to the gynaecologist. Finally, he could no longer control himself when, after all this time, he was told that at their last appointment the doctor had told them, with his usual calm and compassion: "I am giving you a referral; if you still want to have a child, you have two choices: donor insemination or adoption." The analyst said angrily that these torturous procedures had lasted long enough, and without further ado gave the young man the name of a renowned fertility specialist who worked at the hospital near his office. The analyst had had the opportunity to observe this man's competence and tact in the past.

This is how things stood for the analyst and his patient that year, at the beginning of winter—now that they had entered time, they might as well keep track of the seasons. An appointment was made with the other doctor; the patient was to see him in a few weeks. But one day, for the first time since he had started to be on time for his sessions, the patient did not keep his appointment with the analyst. Strangely, he did not even phone to cancel or to explain. This absence constituted a noteworthy event.

A few days later, he arrived exactly on time. The analyst thought he looked strange: fear was again in his eyes. Without a word about his missed appointment, he sat down and started to speak. He and his companion had given refuge in their home to a woman friend in distress, whom they had known for a long time. This friend felt she was losing her wits, after a recent abortion. Lately, she had often told them that she was determined to have a child. When she was pregnant, her partner had violently abused her and forced her to end her pregnancy. The doctors had told her that, for reasons which she seemed unable to remember, she would never be able to have a child. Stalked and threatened by her former partner, she was in a great turmoil and spoke constantly of suicide. The young man and his companion decided to offer her shelter in their home. She arrived with her two dogs, a German shepherd and a poodle.

He described the poodle as a frenetic animal, climbing the walls and pulling on the drapes, while the German shepherd was calm and serene. So this young woman had been living with them for a few days; they treated her with kindness and warmth. Their hospitality probably kept her out of the psychiatric hospital.

And then, two days ago, on the evening before the day when the analyst waited for him in vain, the patient had received a phone call. They were all there, in his living room: the young man, his companion, their friend, and the two dogs. The call was from his sister, who had a baby a few months earlier. She knew they were hoping to have a baby themselves and came straight to the point: "Look, I am sorting through things. I have a bunch of baby clothes to give away. Tell me if the two of you want them."

As he is standing there, the young man realises that he cannot continue this conversation, with this friend sitting across from him, still shaken by her abortion and aware that she can never have children. His companion, next to him, would not have understood how he could have a cryptic conversation about this subject under the circumstances. So he said nothing else and promised to call his sister later. As a result, he was the only one who knew what had been said on the telephone. His companion, their friend, and the two dogs had only been unconscious witnesses—in the narrowest sense of the word: unaware of what had transpired, since they could neither hear nor infer what was said based on his end of the conversation.

He hung up and, a little later, went upstairs with his companion to retire for the night. It was only then that he told her about his sister's call. They decided not to anticipate, and to let things take their course. His sister could keep her baby clothes, they would see about that when their baby would be born. They would not get baby clothes before they had a baby!

The next day, he went to work and did not come home until evening. At this point in his story, his eyes were wide with fear. Night had fallen, it was December. He was coming closer to the house. Usually, when he came home, lights were on and his companion was already there, especially since their friend was staying with them. But now the house was in darkness. He opened the garden gate; he expected to hear the dogs bark as usual. But he heard nothing. He told himself that there was no one home, and that their friend must be out walking the dogs. But terror is present in what he is saying.

In any case, the analyst is gripped with fear, as the atmosphere of the story is transmitted to him directly. The young man continues: he turns the lights on inside; no one is there. He shudders. Like in a Hitchcock movie, there is a hint of something ominous, but everything is normal … Just to be sure, he goes upstairs to see if anyone is home. He goes up the white staircase; the doors of the three bedrooms are closed: obviously, the house is empty. As he comes back down, he notices a small red stain on one of the stairs. Someone must have dropped a marker pen. He gets a wet sponge to wipe away the stain.

The stain disappears easily. But he notices another one, and then another. He follows the trail. It leads to one of the bedrooms. He opens the door. The German shepherd quickly runs out. At the foot of the bed, the poodle lies dead, slaughtered, in a pool of blood. As he finished telling his story, the young man's eyes were popping out of his head, he was scared to death. He just sat there motionless and silent, still seeing the horrific scene imprinted on his retina. As for the two friends, they soon came back from a food-shopping expedition.

In the analyst's office, the end of the story was also followed by an eerie silence, of which the analyst was keenly aware. He heard himself say: "It's the first time a German shepherd does my work for me: he killed the ghost of a dead child by sacrificing the dog that had taken the place of an impossible baby." And he added, remembering his recent conversation with his Swiss colleague Gaetano Benedetti from Bâle: "You know, if it had been the living room clock that had fallen on the dog, I would have said the same thing. The clock could have done my work just as well."

Again, time had made a surreptitious entrance thanks to the illustration chosen by the analyst. In any case, it was clear from the young man's expression and his posture that he was starting to relax. This story was never mentioned again in subsequent sessions with the analyst.

By retelling such a story, the analyst could be taken for an unconditional fan of horror literature, an admirer of E. T. A. Hoffmann, or an unrepentant reader of Jean Ray. But the suspense would have been lost if there had been no need to confirm in what manner time had set itself in motion again, once and for all, on this occasion. Let us say first that the appointment with the fertility specialist recommended by the analyst took place a few days later. The doctor diagnosed bilateral varicocele right away: enlarged veins and raised temperature in the testicles, reducing fertility. The problem could be solved by a simple surgical procedure, which would be performed shortly. But it was very cold that day. The young man had walked to the analyst's office, then to the hospital, and back to his house, covering several kilometres on foot across Paris. In any case, that night, according to the calendar and to the young man's account, a child was conceived, a child that had come from the cold and would arrive exactly nine months later, to everyone's delight.

The young man had the simple surgical procedure performed while his companion was pregnant. Two years after the birth of the first baby, a second child was born, as they had planned; they had been able to leave behind this prehistory in which the young man had almost let himself drown.

And at his side, had the analyst truly abolished the time of death into which he could have been drawn? Had they fought together, as modern incarnations of Don Quixote and Sancho Panza, against the nefarious giants of ordinary perversion? Against what, against whom, had they fought this battle with the help of gods and dogs?

Intellectual tools

First of all, against set formulas. When the two-faced barber asks Don Quixote "not to be vexed", the knight replies: "As to whether I ought to be vexed or not, I myself am the best judge" (De Cervantes, 1605/1615, p. 407).

This is the start of a long preparation for the two heroes before they confront perversion head on. No one can tell Don Quixote how to behave or how to feel. Despite claims of joking and reluctant retractions like "I did not mean it in that way [...], my intention was good", his determination remains steadfast. The curate quickly recognises the theoretical level to which Don Quixote raises the discussion; as a result, he shifts from carrying on an *ad hominem* attack to delivering an historical critique. The reader is advised to consult the classical texts.

To the scholarly question of what credence should be given to the fact that knights-errant "were really and truly persons of flesh and blood" or "fiction, fable and falsehood, and dreams told by men awakened from sleep", Don Quixote replies as Socrates replied to Phaedrus in the dialogue of that name:

> The two men are sitting on a riverbank, near an altar erected to Boreas, the wind, on the spot where thegod carried off the nymph Orythia. Phaedrus asks his master if he believes in these allegories. Socrates answers that a young maid could have fallen while playing on the rocks, pushed off by the wind. But he prefers to believe popular tradition: "If, like the wise men of our day, I don't believe in these stories, I wouldn't be so out of place. [...] All those non-believers [...] will need a great deal of free time. But for me there's no such leisure. And, my dear friend, the reason is this: I am still not able to 'know myself', as the Delphic inscription enjoins, and it seems laughable for me to think about other things when I am still ignorant about myself. So leaving those matters aside, I believe what people say these days ..."
>
> (Plato, c. 370 BC)

In the same way, Cervantes attacks the prejudices of today's learned men who praise positivism. Yet his reader Auguste Comte, the inventor of this principle, agrees with him. Much to the annoyance of his disciples, he credits the "cerebral crisis" he suffered in the spring of 1826 (Gouhier, 1997, p. 149) with the foundation of his theory.

After being hospitalised in Dr Esquirol's clinic for eight months, he decided to leave and gradually recovered, "despite" the ministrations of the famous doctor and "a disastrous drug therapy", but above all thanks to *Don Quixote*, the only book to outline "a true theory of madness before any biologist" (Arbousse-Bastide, 1972, p. 52), a theory that links "the excessive subjectivity of madness" to historical positivity.

We do not intend to contradict Auguste Comte, even though he prefers to speak of synthesis rather than of analysis. The suppression of the links between history and madness, he predicted, would lead to "the fascination with the objective", and "to the error of doctrinal materialism" where transference and speech no longer hold a place.

How, then, can we escape the fascination of the objective and the doctrinal materialism in which we have been ensnared for over a century? Cervantes had already provided an answer when his son delivered a lecture on the psychotherapeutic use of history. To answer the curate's question about fiction and fable, Don Quixote invokes a positive fact, and a double negation.

It is impossible to assert that "knights-errant [...] ever lived in the world". Nor is it possible to draw up a list of references attesting, for example, to the existence of Roland, Charlemagne's nephew. The reader is asked to stand "upon the shoulders of the truth", and to demonstrate an imaginative aptitude. "I can almost say I have with my own eyes seen Amadis of Gaul" (De Cervantes, 1605/1615, p. 407).

Just as Michelet had "almost" seen Joan of Arc (Michelet, 1957), or Jacques Le Goff had almost seen Saint Louis (Le Goff, 2009), by dint of constantly portraying them in the biographies they were writing. Similarly, an analyst trained by Benedetti could "almost" say that he played the role of Neptune in order to fight the fires and draught which Jupiter had inflicted on various regions of the planet. The "almost" defines the potential and transitional space characteristic of children's play, without which, Winnicott tells us, no human endeavour, whether artistic or scientific, could be accomplished:

> I am claiming that these same phenomena that are life and death to our schizoid or borderline patients appear in our cultural experiences. [...] I am assuming that cultural experiences are in direct continuity with play, the play of those who have not yet heard of games.
>
> (Winnicott, 1971, p. 100)

It was this assertion that impelled Niels Bohr, one of the inventors (with Erwin Schrödinger) of quantum mechanics, to tell a young researcher that his theory was not crazy enough. Not to the exclusion of a critical faculty, of course. Don Quixote himself remains realistic in his assertions: "With regard to giants, opinions differ as to whether there ever were any or not in the world."

And he goes on to discuss the very large bones recently discovered in Sicily, which would long continue to fuel archaeological debate. In conclusion, he refers back to "the famous Ariosto" who ended the first book of his adventures by leaving it to others to praise Lady Angelica, of whom: "Some bard of defter quill may sing some day" (De Cervantes, 1605/1615, p. 408).

Here, the two novels intersect beautifully. For what, in fact, is history without its epic cycles, its sagas, and its poems? What would become of deeds and their minute details without the wit which reveals them and recounts them in transference to one who is interested in them?

Soon, Carrasco, the student, launches another surreptitious attack to demolish the knight's ingenuity "it is one thing to write as a poet, another to write as a historian".

What he is insinuating is that Don Quixote is not an historian any more than I am a psychoanalyst, or a sociologist, or my mother's daughter when she said I was not, and so on. Indeed, before his young reader Descartes, at the time still a schoolboy at La Flèche College, wrote "*larvatus prodeo*, on the stage of the world, I advance masked", Cervantes, behind the mask of Don Quixote, scrutinises the professions Freud considered impossible: to educate, to govern, to psychoanalyse. The knight adds: to marry and to publish. He starts by criticising all-powerful marketing that produces "books broadcast on the world as if they were fritters" (De Cervantes, 1605/1615, p. 418).

The high-wire act between reason and madness culminates in high-jinks portraying a topsy-turvy world. Don Quixote imagines himself giving the beautiful Angelica the spanking she deserves for having "turned the world upside down". He speculates that "if Sacripante or Roland had been poets they would have given the damsel a trimming" (De Cervantes, 1605/1615, p. 408).

Now, Sancho Panza, in the title role of the *gracioso*, makes a tumultuous entrance on the stage of this theatre of fools. Shouts are heard outside Don Quixote's door: "at this moment they heard the housekeeper and the niece, who had previously withdrawn from the conversation, exclaiming aloud in the courtyard" (De Cervantes, 1605/1615, p. 409).

With hue and cry, they were announcing the arrival of the clown on the scene of the book, and trying to stop him, while Don Quixote was ordering them to let him in.

The cry of Mother Folly

In France, at the end of the Middle Ages, the Sotties (Aubailly, 1984) put tyrants on trial, not to make them descend "into their coffins", as we sing in the Marseillaise, and set off the vicious cycle of slaying again, but in order to strip them bare. Under the trappings of prestige was revealed the fool's costume, carefully hidden. By contrast, the powerful cry of Mother Folly, which introduces all Sotties, breaks out in full view of everyone present, to summon *graciosos*, fools, and jesters, also called her henchmen. Designated only by numbers, they spill onto the stage gesticulating, to regenerate psyches exhausted by petty and great tyrants alike.

Cervantes forewarned us: here, the text is made of the same fabric, with different designs. As the sottie proceeds, Sancho—Fool number 1, is soon followed by Sanson Carrasco—Fool number 2—then in chapter V by Teresa Panza with her loud mouth—Fool number 3. Carrasco is a blunderer, a mountebank: "he was of no great bodily size, but he as a very great wag; he was of a sallow complexion, but very sharp-witted, somewhere about four-and-twenty years of age, with a round face, a flat nose, and a large mouth, all indications of a mischievous disposition and a love of fun and jokes" (De Cervantes, 1605/1615, p. 414).

Determined to take to the road again, Don Quixote has broken away from his two guardians and set off alone with Sancho in order to recreate the plural body, disbanded a month earlier. The team of caregivers is left with nothing else to do but eavesdrop to find out what they are up to: "I promise you", said the curate, "the niece or the housekeeper will tell us by-and-by, for they are not the ones to forget to listen".

Hush, hush! The mission with which Cervantes entrusted us is still secret. The first exchange between Don Quixote and Sancho Panza concerns the classical topic of the head and the limbs, and asserts their cohesion through the repetition of "together" and "the same". Sancho takes this opportunity to express his usual grievance about the blanketing incident: "when I was blanketed as a member, my head was on the other side of the wall, looking on while I was flying through the air, and did not feel any pain whatever" (De Cervantes, 1605/1615, p. 411).

But Don Quixote doesn't want to keep rehashing the past. What he most urgently desires is to regain access to the outside world, from which he has been cut off for too long, and to set out on a new adventure.

We are familiar with the query he addresses to Sancho, since we learned it by heart as schoolchildren, when we recited Molière:

> Harpagon: And I would know from you, Master Jacques, what it is that is said of me.

> Master Jacques: Yes, certainly, Sir, if I were sure you would not get angry with me.
>
> Harpargon: No, no; never fear.
>
> Master Jacques: Since you wish it, Sir, I will tell you frankly that you are the laughing-stock of everybody. […] You are the butt and jest and byword of everybody …
>
> (Molière, 2004, p. 147)

Molière, Cervantes' reader and disciple, plagiarised his master unabashedly when he too set out on the war path against perversion.

> Don Quixote: "Tell me, Sancho, my friend, what do they say about me in the village here? What do the common people think of me? […] How do they treat the task I have undertaken in reviving and restoring to the world the now forgotten order of chivalry? […] I would have thee tell me […] without adding anything to the good or taking away anything from the bad; for it is the duty of loyal vassals to tell the truth to their lords."
>
> Sancho: "That I will do with all my heart, provided your worship will not be vexed at what I say."
>
> Don Quixote: "I will not be vexed at all, thou mayest speak freely, Sancho."
>
> Sancho: "Well then, first of all, I have to tell you that the common people consider your worship a mighty great madman, and me no less a fool."
>
> (De Cervantes, 1605/1615, p. 412)

Twelve thousand volumes (De Cervantes, 1605/1615, p. 432) of the first novel are sold throughout the world, as many as the bestseller written by Cervantes' master Erasmus, *The Praise of Folly*, which asserts: "The cleverest character in a comedy is the clown, for he who would make people take him for a fool, must not be one" (De Cervantes, 1605/1615, p. 412).

Indeed! By making itself be taken for madness, Folly restores the truth of history eradicated by denial. "History is in a measure a sacred thing, for it should be true."

In truth, Don Quixote learns that after having dubbed himself a knight at the start of the first book, he has acquired great fame, with no need for any publicity or advertising campaign. Cervantes secretly counts on him to avenge his honour as a writer, but does not inform him of this.

Unaware of its ultimate mission, the transferential quartet is coming together, with historical truth playing the role of Dulcinea this time. A signal is all that's needed for it to set off.

Kledôn: *signal for departure*

The sudden neighings of Rocinante and the even louder farts emitted by Dapple punctuate the quartet's desire to set off. This *kledôn*—the name once given to a signal from the Greek gods—was deemed by Don Quixote to be "a happy omen, and he resolved to make another sally in three or four days from that time" (De Cervantes, 1605/1615, p. 422). He encouraged Sancho to keep nurturing the hope that "heaven would make him a fair offer of an island" (De Cervantes, 1605/1615, p. 422).

The second *Don Quixote* gradually exposes the political sequelae of traumas. The departure takes place in the strictest secrecy: a journey to Toboso, to Dulcinea's castle, seat of the knight's symbolic power. In addition, the social link has to be re-established, and nothing is more useful than reflecting on the structures of kinship. The matrimonial plans being elaborated by Sancho and his wife Teresa provide a perfect occasion for this.

Laurence Sterne, a fervent disciple of Cervantes, was to comment later that life is an eternal domestic dispute. For Sancho Panza, the bone of contention this time is the marriage of his daughter Sanchica, "now that she is full-fifteen" (De Cervantes, 1605/1615, p. 425) and having to be preserved from what might well happen unless a husband is quickly found for her. Sancho wants to make a countess of her, while Teresa wants to spare her the humiliation suffered by the "duchess in clogs" the three captains called "villain" (reference to an old French song about the Duchess Ann of Brittany who became queen of France in 1491). She would rather see her daughter marry Lope Tocho, a young fellow from the village, one of her own sort. Sancho will not bend, for he counts on his grandchildren to pull him out of the mire.

The spouses are caught in a fierce class struggle and a merciless battle between the sexes. Having been called an "animal" and an "idiot", Teresa has recourse to the unfailing strategy of beginning "to weep in earnest", stammering between sobs: "The day that I see her a countess, it will be the same to me as if I was burying her; but once more I say do as you please, for we women are born to this burden of being obedient to our husbands, though they be dogs" (De Cervantes, 1605/1615, p. 428).

Teresa's feminist indictment allows her to score a point; Sancho promises to put off as long as possible making Sanchica a countess. Then, convinced that he can entrust the running of his family to his wife's matriarchal authority, he leaves his home, certain that in his absence his children will be safe. At the same time, Don Quixote frees himself from the hold of his niece and his housekeeper, who are, at length, swayed by his arguments. He even gives the housekeeper a lesson in political science: "There is a great difference between … the courtiers who range the world over by looking at a map, and true knights-errant. We, the true knights-errant, are exposed to the sun, to the cold, to the air …; nor do we only know enemies in pictures, but in their own real shapes" (De Cervantes, 1605/1615, p. 429–430).

The knight realises that his young niece takes him for an old fogy when she reels off the discourse of the barber and the curate: "all this you are saying about knights-errant is fable and fiction; and their histories … would deserve, each of them, to have a *sambenito* put on it …, if indeed they were not burned" (De Cervantes, 1605/1615, p. 430).

The tone of the young lass has the ring of indoctrination. Therefore, her uncle puts her in her place: "Can it be that a young hussy that hardly knows how to handle a dozen lace-bobbins dares to wag her tongue and criticize the histories of knights-errant?" (De Cervantes, 1605/1615, p. 430).

And, to dissuade her from holding forth on anything and everything, he delivers an analysis worthy of Wittgenstein: "To understand a language is to be master of a technique … through example. It is a practice" (1953, paragraph 199). According to Don Quixote: "nor is it everyone that calls himself a gentleman, that is so in all respects; some are gold, others pinchbeck, and all look like gentlemen, but not all can stand the touchstone of truth" (De Cervantes, 1605/1615, p. 431).

Then he goes on at length to lecture his "young hussy" of a niece on lineages, the practice of generosity, and the transmission of names—spheres in which there "is great confusion", since, to quote Wittgenstein again, "giving a thing a name is not like attaching a label to a thing" (1953), just as the three letters of the title "Do not guarantee superior character"; without virtue and generosity, "a great man who is vicious will be a great example of vice …; for the possessor of wealth is not made happy by possessing it, but by spending it, and not by spending as he pleases, but by knowing how to spend it well" (De Cervantes, 1605/1615, p. 432).

The spending of which Don Quixote speaks is not that associated with consumerism. Akin to the practice of *potlatch* and to the "give away" of the Amerindians, its goal is to reinitiate the social link by taking care "not to mix sacred things with profane". Don Quixote insists that it is important to tread the path of virtue rather than to go down "the broad and easy road of vice which ends in death" (De Cervantes, 1605/1615, p. 432). He even draws on an elegy by the poet Garcilaso de la Vega to make his point.

The young girl is very impressed: "Woe is me!" exclaimed the niece, "my lord is a poet, too! He knows everything, and he can do everything; ... he could make a house as easily as a cage."

The lass has just seen her uncle escape with head held high from the cage to which self-appointed judges had confined him. Certain that nothing could be expected of him, they speculated on the uselessness of his unworthiness. But they were wrong: "I can tell you, niece, ... there would be nothing that I could not do, not any sort of knickknack that would not come from my hands, particularly cages and toothpicks" (De Cervantes, 1605/1615, p. 433).

Indeed, the second novel gradually constructs the cage that will serve to entrap the deadly intentions which threaten the novel itself. In order to draw up a plan, Don Quixote withdraws to his room with Sancho, to organise a third sally. Alarmed, the housekeeper goes off to find the bachelor Sanson Carrasco, and shouts: "... my master is breaking out, he is ... breaking out at the door of his madness" (De Cervantes, 1605/1615, p. 434).

In truth, nothing can stop the transferential quartet now, not even the fierce contract negotiations undertaken by Sancho to obtain higher wages and a risk premium, on Teresa's advice, since "a woman's advice is no great thing, and he who won't take it is a fool" (De Cervantes, 1605/1615, p. 435).

His master is not intimidated by the threat of a strike. Taking advantage of the situation, the student tries to take control by intervening in the argument between master and squire, on the pretext of resolving their differences. By no means fooled by his intervention, Don Quixote lets Sancho believe that "the perpetual joy and delight of the courts of the Salamancan schools" could indeed make a suitable squire, though it would be a shame to endanger "this pillar of letters and vessel of the sciences, and cut down this towering palm of the fair and liberal arts" (De Cervantes, 1605/1615, p. 438).

This initial crisis reinforces the alliance between Don Quixote and Sancho. The latter agrees to stop "bargaining more or less" about his wages: "it was only to please my wife …; but after all, a man must be a man, and a woman a woman" (De Cervantes, 1605/1615, p. 438).

Following these words of wisdom, the two heroes embrace one another, while the bachelor looks on in amazement. The plural body is reinforced and the departure is planned for three days thence. In the meantime, we have learned that Sancho's loyalty to the knight is not total, and that the affection between them (*philia*) is far from ideal.

Don Quixote and Sancho sally forth

The two mounts, the horse and the donkey, give the departure signal: "the moment Sanson took his departure, Rocinante began to neigh, and Dapple to sigh" (De Cervantes, 1605/1615, p. 440), which means to pass wind. The Moorish historian Cide Hamete salutes the start of the adventure with a solemn "Blessed be Allah the all-powerful!" This time, the destination is not the plains of Montiel, but rather El Toboso, the region where Don Quixote's Lady is to join the transferential procession; the Lady must always be reconquered and saved from the defamation inflicted on Don Quixote and his creator.

On the journey, the talking cure is taken up again, in the same manner as in the first novel, on the endless question of evidence for the existence of Dulcinea (De Cervantes, 1605/1615, p. 221). Neither of the heroes has actually seen her, although Sancho continues to pretend that he has seen her sifting wheat in a cloud of dust, while his master maintains that she was stringing pearls.

Be that as it may, the important thing is to call forth the Lady again, in "some rich and royal palace" (De Cervantes, 1605/1615, p. 441), the "interior castle", as Saint Teresa of Avila (Allendesalazar, 2002, p. 2) called it, located at the bottom of the Lake of Boiling Pitch.

Cervantes' need for the Lady is particularly great since, as he embarks upon the writing of the second novel, he must withstand the deadly attacks of forgers and "the spite which some wicked enchanter seems to have against everything of mine", in Don Quixote's words. Soon, a real castle will materialise where envy acts as a "cankerworm" of the social link (De Cervantes, 1605/1615, p. 441), "pressing men against each other" (Arendt, 1951), as Hanna Arendt puts it.

To illustrate his point, the knight tells Sancho a story. A poet wrote a satire against all the courtesan ladies. One of them, insulted not to have been named specifically, threatened him unless he added her name to the list. The poet consented, and "left her without a shred of reputation". Having made the headlines of the scandal sheets, the lady "was satisfied by getting fame though it was infamy" (De Cervantes, 1605/1615, p. 442).

The story seems trivial today, when advertising agencies specialise in procuring fame without destroying the Temple of Diana in Ephesus, or burning the Golden Pavilion in Kyoto (Mishima, 1959), as was done long ago, "with the sole object of making one's name live in after ages". Interestingly, although Sancho and his master are very concerned with the ages to come, they are not concerned with any popularity rating: "while I see myself put into a book and passed on from hand to hand over the world, I don't care a fig, let them say what they like of me" (De Cervantes, 1605/1615, p. 442).

How, then, are we to distinguish between acquiring a good name and leading a publicity campaign? While the heroes are spending the night on the edge of a wood, we learn about their battle plan: they will burst narcissistic pride by slaying giants, and overcome "envy by generosity and nobleness of heart, anger by calmness of demeanor and equanimity, ... lust and lewdness by the loyalty we preserve to ... the mistresses of our thoughts, indolence by traversing the world" (De Cervantes, 1605/1615, p. 443). To pass one's name down to future centuries is no easy task. One must cross "the dark night" (*noche oscura*) of St John of the Cross, whose funeral procession we have already encountered in the first novel (De Cervantes, 1605/1615, p. 112). Now, Sancho knows what they have to do: "let us set about becoming saints", he tells his master.

The *Spiritual Canticle*, written by St John of the Cross in Cervantes' time, is not devoid of Quixotic accents. They are particularly clear in the "Song of the Soul", in which the Soul (*el Alma*), sings to her bridegroom Christ:

> In search of my Love
> I will go over mountains and strands;
> I will gather no flowers,
> I will fear no wild beasts;
> And pass by the mighty and the frontiers.
>
> (St John of the Cross, 1585, p. 9)

When dark night fell over the city of El Toboso, the two heroes left the woods and were assailed, like in the previous adventure of the fulling hammers (De Cervantes, 1605/1615, p. 117), by sounds at once familiar and frightening: "Now and then an ass brayed, pigs grunted, cats mewed, and the various noises they made seemed louder in the silence of the night; all which the enamored knight took to be of evil omen" (De Cervantes, 1605/1615, p. 446).

They are off to a bad start, and the worst is yet to come. The worst is the twisted plan devised by Sancho—that most loyal of men—based on "the falsehood of the reply he had brought [Don Quixote] in the Sierra Morena on behalf of Dulcinea". The small lie in the First Part will reach uncontrollable proportions in the Second Part.

At the end of a soliloquy in which Sancho reflects on ways of getting out of this second embassy to Dulcinea, he makes up a story that he has seen her changed into a peasant girl on a she-ass, riding in the company of two friends.

Compelled to kneel down in order to pay his respects to the peasant girl, Don Quixote remained "with his eyes starting out of his head [at] a village lass, and not a very well-favored one, for she was platter-faced and snub-nosed", and took him for the sort of fellow village girls have learned to mistrust: "See how the lordlings come to make game of the village girls now. ... Hey-day! My grandfather! Much I care for your lovemaking!" (De Cervantes, 1605/1615, p. 453).

No sooner has she sped away than she fell off her reluctant mount; she then "took a short run, and ... dropped into the saddle more lightly than a falcon, and sat astride like a man". Don Quixote's mistrust of his own perceptions resembles the stupefaction he felt when the room where he kept his library was walled up unbeknownst to him, after the burning of his books (De Cervantes, 1605/1615, p. 40).

A word to the wise! The "hypocrite reader" is given fair warning. No monkey business, or Cervantes will count him among the enchanters who pursue him and his son with their "malice and spite".

Polyphonies

Now renowned throughout Europe, Don Quixote is less given to undertaking actions that might propel him through the looking glass. But this new attitude does not protect him from anxiety. On the verge of making his third sally, he is suddenly gripped with fright.

Always faithful to his duties, despite his lies, Sancho continues to act as a *therapon*:

> cheer up that little heart of yours, master mine, for at the present moment you seem to have got one no bigger than a hazelnut; remember what they say, that a stout heart breaks bad luck, ... and moreover they say, the hare jumps up where it's not looked for.
>
> (De Cervantes, 1605/1615, p. 450)

Like on a medieval wall tapestry on which the hare suddenly springs into view, Sancho's proverbs, interspersed in the text, resonate like Villon's "The Ballad of Proverbs": "We call out Christmas till 'tis here" (Villon, 1489c, Vol. X, pp. 15–17), or his *Ballade*: "I know everything but myself." Words thrown in by the squire at random, such as: "the truth may run fine but will not break, and always rises above falsehood as oil above water" (De Cervantes, 1605/1615, p. 449)—play the same role as the Greek *kledônes* (Flacelière, 1965). These involuntary interjections considered oracular often spring from the mouths of fools, simpletons, or children.

Such an omen occurs when the heroes encounter "The Cortes of Death", a religious play attributed to Lope de Vega, presented by a travelling theatre. This scene foreshadows Don Quixote's death, and the loss of Dulcinea—announced in the Prologue to the Second Part.

Dating back to Monteverdi's era, Dulcinea gradually becomes the harmonic tone of the Cervantian oeuvre, which makes the souls of readers vibrate century after century, long after the end of the second novel, when Don Quixote's soul is called back to its dwelling place.

The theatre of death

Don Quixote leaves El Toboso with a heavy heart. Rocinante, his bridle dangling from his neck, testifies to the knight's dejection. Sancho, the mischief-maker, continues to provide moral bolstering: "control yourself, your worship, be yourself again; gather up Rocinante's reins .... What the devil is this? What weakness is this? Are we here or in France?"

Was France already renowned for its depression? Don Quixote's reaction is to take responsibility for the situation, just as children, and even babies, do when their trust has been betrayed. "Hush, Sancho, ... and utter no blasphemies against that enchanted lady; for I alone am to blame for her misfortune and hard fate; her calamity has come of the hatred the wicked bear me."

Here, the delusion is aimed at the part of the truth that survives the lie; Cervantes will use all kinds of theatrical forms to enact this truth. After having "presented", in the First Part of the novel, the unspeakable traumas of his father's war and captivity, Don Quixote can now "represent" the truth that survives perversion.

On a cart, "Death itself with a human face" (De Cervantes, 1605/1615, p. 457) appears before him. But he quickly checks his impulse to attack, when the leader of the procession informs him that they are actors in a travelling theatre company. The first thing the knight does is to pay tribute to actors, voicing the author's love for theatre: "God speed you, good people, keep your festival ..., for from a child I was fond of the play, and in my youth a keen lover of the actor's art" (De Cervantes, 1605/1615, p. 458).

From a child! Since then, Cervantes must have become disillusioned. Although he wrote plays when he returned from Algiers, the ones he authored after the success of *Don Quixote* were never performed. Now, he has a score to settle with theatre people, and he proceeds to do so through a fourth story of fools, as ferocious as the ones he told before.

Popping up suddenly like a jack-in-the-box, one of the actors "in a mummer's dress with a great mummer of bells" makes his appearance. True to the etymology of the word "folly"—*follis*, bellows full of air—he is "armed with three blown ox bladders at the end of a stick", which he shakes with a "great jingling of bells". The knight is suddenly less enthusiastic. Seeing "this merry-andrew ... banging the ground with the bladders and cutting capers", Rocinante was startled, took the bit between his teeth, and sped off, throwing his rider to the ground. Worse still, when Sancho jumped off Dapple to rescue his master, "the dancing devil" jumped upon the ass and flew across the fields, until he was thrown off in his turn.

It's time to speak frankly to "actors ... of the royal companies", who are protected even when they commit crimes. As violent as the convicts in the first novel, they are ready to attack him with "a mighty discharge of stones", after hearing the insults delivered by Don Quixote on Cervantes' behalf, "even if the whole human race favors them" (De Cervantes, 1605/1615, p. 459).

The encounter with the Cortes of Death illustrates the scorn of Cervantes' enemies who had announced his Dulcinea's downfall, since indeed many of his works for the stage were lost. Based on the few plays that survived—as well as on short "interludes" (Marrast, 1983)—Jean Canavaggio shows that Cervantes' theatre was clearly ahead of its time (1977).

But no matter! Banished from the stage, his theatrical genius makes a triumphant comeback in the second novel, taking on all possible forms of the "mirror of comedy" which act as "instruments of great good to the State, [showing] us more faithfully what we are".

"Sotties", farces, and morality plays, musical comedies, puppet shows, baroque theatre, opera, and oratorios are all staged in succession up to the knight's death throes, enacted on the model of Socrates' death (Plato, c. 370 BC).

Fools and knaves

Having triumphed over the false friends who had vowed to do him in, Cervantes pays homage to the *philia* between Rocinante and Dapple.

> Between [them] there was a friendship so unequalled [that] the two beasts would eagerly scratch one another when they were together and ... when they were tired and full, Rocinante would lay his neck across Dapple's, stretching half a yard or more on the other side, and the pair would stand thus, gazing thoughtfully on the ground, for three days.
>
> (De Cervantes, 1605/1615, p. 462)

The author likens them to Orestes and Pylades; they illustrate the paradigm of the plural body of survival, "to the admiration of mankind ..., shaming men, who preserve friendship with one another so badly". The novel is undeniably infused with an animist spirit. "And let no one fancy that the author was at all astray when he compared the friendship of these animals to that of men, for men have received many lessons from beasts."

Indeed, a false friend promptly makes his appearance in the flashy shape of Sanson Carrasco disguised as Knight of the Mirrors, with his pseudo Lady, Casildea de Vandalia, and his pseudo squire named the Squire of the Grove, who sports a huge false nose. The student's intention is to make the knight see reason, so that he can insinuate himself in this prestigious tale, displacing the barber and the curate and gaining fame, "though it [be] infamy".

Less naive than his master, Sancho boasts of coming from a Panza line of wine-tasters who could detect the presence of a rusty key with its leather thong in a cask of wine (De Cervantes, 1605/1615, pp. 470–471). Like his ancestor, he detects the ruse and stands firm: "I have spoken—it only makes it worse to stir it" (De Cervantes, 1605/1615, p. 465).

When the long-nosed squire declares that his master is "more roguish than crazy or valiant", Sancho responds by painting a portrait of his own master worthy of the great Fra Angelico:

> Mine is not that [...], he has the soul of a pitcher; he has no thought of doing harm to anyone, only good to all, nor has he any malice whatever in him; a child might persuade him that it is night at noonday; and for this simplicity I love him as the core of my heart, and I can't bring myself to leave him, let him do ever such foolish things.
>
> (De Cervantes, 1605/1615, p. 469)

We imagine the little band fluttering like birds around St Francis of Assisi and Saint Clara, his Dulcinea, in Rossellini's *The Flowers of St Francis*. Now, *fools* and *knaves* are clearly opposed. Swift may have remembered the Fioretti in his "Digression on madness", when he spoke of wishing to reach "the sublime and refined point of felicity, called the possession of being well deceived, the serene peaceful state of ... being a *fool* among knaves" (Swift, 1704).

By inventing a virtual story to fascinate and disorient the heroes, Carrasco forces his way into Don Quixote's story. The resemblance to the forger who usurped the first novel is certainly not fortuitous: "What I most ... pride myself upon is having vanquished in single combat that so famous knight Don Quixote of La Mancha ..., and ... his glory, his fame, and his honor have passed and are transferred to my person" (De Cervantes, 1605/1615, p. 473).

Today, the procedure has been patented all over the world, as neurologist Antonio Damasio confirms. To explain our transformation into zombies wavering between violence and lethargy, there is no need to invoke "misery or neurotransmitters, any more than legal or illegal drugs" (Damasio, 2005). All that is needed is to confuse our perceptions and replace them with sham discernment. Hannah Arendt used the term "fictitious" to describe the "ice cold reasoning" which classifies all opponents to the regime as feeble-minded (1951), or leads to even worse measures.

But Don Quixote, who has recovered from his father's trauma, can no longer be tricked. Instead of falling into the trap, he took the time to have an internal monologue and "he restrained himself as well as he could, in order to force [Sanson Carrasco] to confess the lie with his own lips" (De Cervantes, 1605/1615, p. 473). He told himself that there is no use arguing with a scoundrel. You smash his face. And that's just what he did, striking the Knight of the Mirrors with great force, and throwing him from his horse.

Don Quixote's victory in the first round is rewarded by "gay-plumaged birds of all sorts [that] began to warble in the trees, and with their varied and gladsome notes seemed to welcome and salute the fresh morn" (De Cervantes, 1605/1615, p. 476). On this enchanted morning, already captured in song forty years earlier by Clément Janequin, Rocinante broke into a gallop "on this occasion only", bearing down on the knight on his sluggish horse, who refused to heed the urging of the spurs.

After "he brought [him] to the ground", Don Quixote could not believe that he was really his "friend, the bachelor Sanson Carrasco". He could not imagine that a friend would stage such a farce. Even when the huge-nosed squire "Tomé Cecial ... gossip and friend of Sancho Panza" (De Cervantes, 1605/1615, p. 479) removed his fake nose in order to be recognised, Don Quixote was not convinced. He refused to believe that a friend can change into an enemy, unless enchanters have gotten into the act.

The workings of the perverse mechanisms which govern "the swinding of thought and the highjacking of intelligence" have been described by Paul-Claude Racamier, whose advice is to stay away from their deathly spheres (1992, p. 295). Cervantes does just the opposite, sending his son right into the fray, to teach us how to detect land mines hidden underground.

The secret of their home-made scheme will only be revealed in the next chapter, in which we learn that a therapeutic psychodrama was elaborated in a "staff meeting", ostensibly for the patient's sake: "it was decided by the unanimous vote of all, ... that Don Quixote should be allowed to go" and resume his pathological journey, knowing that the bachelor Sanson would be sent to bring him back, arranging "to meet him [dressed] as a knight-errant". In the event that the scheme was successful, "the bachelor knight was to command him to return to his village and his house, and not quit it for two years; ... and during the period of his seclusion he might perhaps forget his folly, or there might be an opportunity of discovering some ready remedy for his madness" (De Cervantes, 1605/1615, p. 481).

New remedies for madness are constantly being sought, since the revelation of the side effects of the latest discovery creates the need for a new one. But this time, the failure of the plotted therapy triggers a caregivers' vendetta, like those often mounted against non-compliant patients. Carrasco's manhunt turns nasty. He confesses to his co-conspirators that "it is not any wish that he may recover his senses that will make me hunt him out now, but a wish for the sore pain I am in with my ribs" (De Cervantes, 1605/1615, p. 482).

At least, his view of caregiving is clear. He does not mince words. The clown has turned into a sinister jokester, the one designated by the title of David Rousset's book *Le pitre ne rit pas* (The Clown Is Not Laughing; 1948) about Nazi atrocities in the Second World War. In these times of Baroque poetry and metamorphoses, Cervantes can see the passage from laughter to terror. The ground of errantry has become slippery. Will the knight identify himself as a victim of persecution and imagine, as Nobel Prize writer Gao Xingjian puts it, "that becoming sacrificed is a great honour"? (2000).

On the contrary, far from cultivating a marginal status and looking for supporters, Don Quixote delivers a discourse on education devoid of any demagogy, to underscore the difference between education and indoctrination.

Education

After the clamour of the duel, Cervantes, a well-versed musician, provides the reader with a space of peace and silence. While the storm clouds of a vendetta are gathering on the horizon unbeknownst to him, Don Quixote is filled with joy and pride because he has been "victorious in the conflict over the perverse enchanter and malignant magicians" (De Cervantes, 1605/1615, pp. 483–484). And yet, the blow to the agency of the Lady, after Sancho's trickery, has been recorded by the seismograph of his soul. Despite the high spirits conferred by his victory, he was filled with a "deep melancholy".

Betrayal by one's own is not confined to wartime, as Sancho has shown. He forced his master to see Dulcinea "in the repulsive and mean form of a coarse country wench, with cloudy eyes and a foul smell in her mouth" (De Cervantes, 1605/1615, p. 484). Did this allow Sancho to gain the upper hand over his master, as was the case in the movie *The Servant* (1963), directed by Joseph Losey?

Sancho knew "that the transformation of Dulcinea has been a device and imposition of his own ..., but he did not like to reply lest he should say something that might disclose his trickery". In the meantime, Don Quixote is left to ponder on what might serve as an explanation for Carrasco's hostility. "Have I ever been by any chance his enemy? Have I ever given him any occasion to owe me a grudge? Am I his rival ...?" (De Cervantes, 1605/1615, p. 483).

Perversion with its speedy attack always counts on a belated reaction on the part of the prey—the time lost in trying to understand why. Taking refuge in the woods again, the knight is trying to rebuild his energy in this liminal space between wilderness and civilisation, so that he may rescue raped maidens, abused widows, and disowned orphans, still very numerous on the planet, despite the efforts of non-profit organisations. Don Quixote's delusion is a lie detector that identifies enchanters as the origin of the deception, who "change one countenance into another, turning fair into foul, and foul into fair".

When a second rider appears on the road, "dressed in an overcoat of fine green cloth [and] mounted on a very handsome dappled mare" (De Cervantes, 1605/1615, p. 484), the reader is propelled into an Arthurian legend, where he comes face to face with the Green Knight. The two riders stared at each other with curiosity. Don Quixote's appearance astonished the man in green, who "struck [the knight] as being a man of intelligence", after he had examined him closely (De Cervantes, 1605/1615, p. 485). Once again, the knight states his name and reports on his reputation, summarising the adventures on which he embarked in the first novel, stepping through the looking glass. Now, he can introduce himself and look at himself in the mirror of chivalry, having no choice but to "sound [his] own praise ... when there is no one at hand to do it for [him]" (De Cervantes, 1605/1615, p. 485).

To complete the portrait of the character he chooses to embody, he adds: "My desire was to bring to life again knight-errantry, now dead, and for some time past, stumbling here, falling there, now coming down headlong, now captaining myself up again, I have carried out a great portion of my design."

His enthusiasm causes him to triple the financial benefit obtained from the sale of his adventures, and he makes a prospective assessment that doctors of his era could rightly have called manic, were it not for the fact that this figure has since been largely exceeded. "I have been already found worthy to make my way in print to well nigh all, or most, of the nations of the earth. Thirty thousand volumes of my history have been printed, and it is on the high road to be printed thirty thousand thousands of times" (De Cervantes, 1605/1615, p. 485).

The knight in the green coat is among those who exchange playfully with Don Quixote, instead of playing games with him. Contrary to Vivaldo, the traveller encountered on the way to Chrysostom's funeral (De Cervantes, 1605/1615, p. 69), Don Diego de Miranda is an "admirable" man who has remained true to ancient traditions, and who welcomes the knight and his squire into his home, where they meet his wife and their only son, Lorenzo, an eighteen-year-old youth. Don Quixote greatly appreciated "the marvelous silence that reigned throughout the house, for it was like a Carthusian monastery" (De Cervantes, 1605/1615, p. 501). As for Sancho, he considered Don Diego a saint.

For the past six years, Lorenzo has been a student in Salamanca. Less self-assured than Carrasco, but by all accounts a good student, the choice of his studies worries his father. Instead of studying in a law school or at the very least in some business school, he insists on becoming a poet. He is fascinated with Latin and Greek authors, as if the Spanish—busy colonising Latin America at the time—were not worthy of his interest. In the course of this conversation, Cervantes has Don Quixote deliver a lesson in educational methods, which the reader is entrusted with delivering to the forger.

First:

> be they good or bad, [children] are to be loved as we love the souls that give us life; it is for the parents to guide them from infancy in their ways of virtue … (;) and to force them to study this or that science. I do not think wise, though it may be no harm to persuade them; … and it would be my advice to them … to let [a child] pursue whatever science [his parents] may see him most inclined to.
>
> (De Cervantes, 1605/1615, pp. 487–488)

The second lesson concerns the protection of the Spanish language, fifty years after the "Defence and Illustration of the French Language" by the literary group "La Pléiade". Don Diego should encourage his son to cultivate his mother tongue, despite a renewed infatuation with Antiquity in the Renaissance.

> I am inclined to think that [your son] is not quite right [...]; in short, all the ancient poets wrote in the language they imbibed with their mother's milk. [...] Poetry, gentle sir, is [...] like a tender young maiden who [...] will not bear to be dragged through the streets. [...] She must not be touched by [...] the ignorant vulgar. [...] And do not suppose, senor, that I apply the term vulgar here merely to plebians and the lower orders, for everyone who is ignorant, be he lord or prince, may and should be included among the vulgar.
>
> (De Cervantes, 1605/1615, p. 488)

The vulgarity of the elite will be exposed before long, in the episode which takes place at the ducal castle. A word to the wise! Hearing this discourse on child education, Don Diego starts to hesiate as to his travelling companion's folly or sanity. The reader will soon be able to decide.

Cheese and neuroscience

A famous illumination seen in the psalm Insipiens (Jéquier, 1993, pp. 43–52) represents the fool holding cheese in his hands. In the twelfth century, Saint Hildegarde explained the meaning of this image through one of her visions, in which souls were differentiated like cheese after refining: well or not so well aged. Cervantes applies the Saint's vision to the white matter of the brain, and provides a "cheese theory" of the psychic apparatus in cases of madness.

Earlier on their journey, Sancho had placed curds in his master's helmet to keep them cool. Don Quixote suddenly donned his helmet and thought that his "head is softening, or [his] brains are melting" when the curds "began to run all over his face and beard" (De Cervantes, 1605/1615, p. 490).

Having been baptised by this "rain of cheese", he can solemnly undertake the mad task of opening the door of the lions' cage on a cart encountered on the road. Two lions, "of enormous size, and grim and hideous mien" (De Cervantes, 1605/1615, p. 494), are in the same position as he had been a month earlier. The totemic illustration is perfect. In fact, as Aby Warburg pointed out, "the domain of mythology is not ruled by the principle of minimum energy. On the contrary, to render things palpable, a being saturated with demonic energy is needed, for a full understanding of the causes of mysterious events" (2015).

Thus, the knight has decided to do battle with the two caged beasts. It is time for him to regain his prestige as Knight of the Sad Countenance, and earn the more aristocratic title of Knight of the Lions. Unable to dissuade him, Sancho, Don Diego, and the carters transporting the lions run away from the cart to avoid witnessing the massacre. The challenge launched to King Noble in the fable of Raynard the Fox (Larned, 1925) is formulated (ironically) by the narrator, in a heroic-comic style:

> On foot, alone, undaunted, high-souled, with but a simple sword, and that no trenchant blade of the Perrillo brand, a shield, but no bright polished steel one, there stoodst thou, biding and awaiting the two fiercest lions that Africa's forests ever bred! … I leave [thy deeds] as they stand, wanting the words wherewith to glorify them!

The scene that follows is reminiscent of the confrontation between two Japanese sabre masters. The lion "stretched himself thoroughly; he next opened his mouth, and yawned very leisurely, and with near two palms' length of tongue that he had thrust forth, he licked the dust out of his eyes and washed his face; having done this, he … looked all around with eyes like glowing coals, a spectacle and demeanor to strike terror into temerity itself". Then, considering the combat useless, either because it was obviously equal or because his enemy was not worth the trouble, he "turned about and presented his hindquarters to Don Quixote, and very coolly and tranquilly lay down again in the cage".

To console Don Quixote, who had been eager for a fight, the keeper of the two lions, acting as referee, declares him victorious and entitled to display tamed lions on his shield, like those on the Dutch coat of arms.

This truce with the space of wilderness allows Don Quixote to free himself elegantly from the sophistry which entraps him, and to finally allow himself some rest in the home of his new host, a "house built in village style". Since the era of the first novel, the quality of accommodations has been much improved. There is room to breathe! But Don Diego, still worried about his son's future, doesn't know what to think. Should he trust the knight's advice or not? He "acts [like] the greatest madman in the world, and [makes] observations so sensible that they efface and undo all he does" (De Cervantes, 1605/1615, p. 499), leaving one to wonder whether he is mad or sane. He entrusts his son with making this difficult decision: "Do thou talk to him and feel the pulse of his wits, and as thou art shrewd, form the most reasonable conclusion thou canst as to his wisdom or folly" (De Cervantes, 1605/1615, p. 499).

Don Quixote does not back down. Freshly bathed and dressed in his best finery, he is ready to combat "triumphant sloth" (De Cervantes, 1605/1615, p. 501) and provide the young man with an encyclopaedic education.

For, indeed, "knight-errantry is a science" which involves the knowledge of justice, theology, medicinal plants, psychotherapy, astronomy to find one's bearings, mathematics, "for at every turn some occasion for them will present itself" (De Cervantes, 1605/1615, p. 500), swimming and the equestrian arts, for knowing how to shoe a horse and repair the saddle and bridle. "You have to be able to swim" is something Martin Cooperman, the psychoanalyst working with psychosis at the Austen Riggs Center, used to say as well. After all, the aircraft carrier Wasp, on which he served as a flight surgeon, was sunk at Guadalcanal in 1942.

Impressed with the knight's erudition, Lorenzo reports to his father that he can draw no conclusion as to their guest's sanity: "All the doctors and clever scribes in the world will not make sense of the scrawl of this madness: he is a madman full of streaks, full of lucid intervals" (De Cervantes, 1605/1615, p. 501), impossible to classify.

Moreover, he does not have the slightest concern about what people say, and thinks that it is better to lose through excess than through deficit. In short, he is "too much"! Enthralled by Don Quixote, the youth asks him to evaluate a commentary in verse that he has written on a four-line riddle: "Could 'was' become an 'is' for me/, Or … the time that is/Become the time that is to be!" (De Cervantes, 1605/1615, p. 502).

Far from being disconcerted, the knight responds with great enthusiasm to Lorenzo's talent: "God knows, I would gladly take Don Lorenzo with me to teach him … virtues that are part and parcel of the profession I belong to; but … his tender age does not allow it, nor his praiseworthy pursuits permit it" (De Cervantes, 1605/1615, p. 504).

Despite his desire to win the young lad over to his cause, Don Quixote decides to take leave, to avoid outstaying his welcome. Some years ago, one could still make out this adage over the door of the guesthouse of the Abbaye of Fontenay in Burgundy: "Fish and guests. Both stink in three days."

Alliances

After acquiring an education, the next stage is that of forming an alliance. This theme might be inspired by Cervantes' troubles with the illegitimate daughter he had with Ana Franca de Rojas before marrying

Catalina de Salazar. Isabel de Saavedra, as she was called, was always trying to assess the benefits she could reap from her husbands. When the wealthy Camacho marries the fair Quiteria, the knight is entrusted with defending Basilio, the poor, rejected suitor.

Don Quixote and Sancho are led to the wedding celebrations by two students encountered on the road, who listened to the knight "with admiration and respect", although they "perceived the crack in Don Quixote's pate". On this occasion, the knight's teaching is delivered in the form of a comparison between marriage and a travelling companion. "[He] who has to make a whole journey of life down to the final halting place of death, will look out for some trusty and pleasant companion to accompany him before he sets out …, more especially when the companion has to be his companion in bed, at board, and everywhere" (De Cervantes, 1605/1615, p. 507).

Indeed, Miguel journeyed with Catalina until his death. Thirty years after their marriage, he was preparing to join her in the Tertiary Order of Saint Francis, into which she had entered with her sister-in-law, Andrea Cervantes. The alliance must triumph over market-value considerations: "The companionship of one's wife is no article of merchandise that … may be returned, or bartered, or changed." Still, the picture of marriage is not entirely idyllic: "it is an inseparable accident that lasts as long as life lasts; it is a noose that, once you put it round your neck, turns into a Gordian knot, which, if the scythe of Death does not cut it, there is no untying".

True to his male bigotry, Sancho explains this state of affairs by saying: "between a woman's 'yes' and 'no' I wouldn't venture to put the point of a pin, for there would not be room for it."

Launching into the recitation of a string of proverbs whose grammar his master has to correct, Sancho is indignant that Don Quixote "is always graveling" at everything he says (De Cervantes, 1605/1615, p. 508), and invokes their agreement, stipulating "that I was to be let say all I liked". Don Quixote cuts him off, saying: "and even if it were so, I desire you to hold your tongue" (De Cervantes, 1605/1615, p. 508).

But speech does not give up so easily, and becomes the damsel for whom duels deserve to be fought. The two students become involved in the dispute. One of them castigates the other, saying: "if you did not pride yourself more on your dexterity with those foils you carry than on dexterity of the tongue, you would have been head of the degrees, where you are now tail" (De Cervantes, 1605/1615, pp. 511–512).

The licentiate, a "master of fence" as skilled as the young Descartes had been, unsheathed his sword on the spot. On guard! When Cervantes left the University of Alcala to go off to fight in Italy, he chose the sword over the study of letters. Meeting these young men on the road was very likely an encounter with his own youth. Once the students reconciled, the field was free for the amorous squirmish centring around fair Quiteria's marriage to the wealthy Camacho, at the expense of the indigent Basilio.

From the edge of the woods where they had spent another night, Don Quixote and Sancho witnessed a splashy spread, making it clear that the future bridegroom's family had spared no expense. The sight produced a profound impression on Sancho: "the best foundation in the world is money. [Would Basilio] be not poor, he would marry Quiteria" (De Cervantes, 1605/1615, p. 511).

Like in a Bruegel painting, the peasant wedding displays, in the foreground, an abundance of wines and victuals. In the background, one can see young sword dancers, revellers dancing jigs to the sound of bagpipes, girls in flowery dresses, and riders galloping on horses with bells. On a higher plane, on raised boards, the figures of Love, Interest, and Poetry are staging morality plays in the midst of wild men accompanied by tabor- and flute-players. Sancho, who has gobbled down a bucket of geese and hens, is now definitely on Camacho's side, prompting his master to say: "It is easy to see thou art a clown, Sancho, and one of the sort that cry 'Long life to the conqueror'" (De Cervantes, 1605/1615, p. 516).

To this, Sancho opposes his grandmother's wisdom: "As much as thou hast so much art thou worth, and as much as thou art worth so much hast thou.... there are only two families in the world, the Haves and the Haven'ts; and she stuck to the Haves."

As for Basilio, to the display of lavish expense, he opposes the ultimate gesture of *seppuku*, committing suicide in the style of Baroque theatre: sword through the body, a flood of blood, contortions, dying words—nothing is neglected, not even the last sacrament of the dying, which Basilio accepts on condition that Quiteria first give him her hand in marriage, before he abandons her to his rival. Sancho alone remains unmoved by all this pathos: "For one so badly wounded, this young man has a great deal to say; they should ... attend to his soul; for to my thinking he has it more on his tongue than between his teeth" (De Cervantes, 1605/1615, p. 521).

Indeed, as soon as the couple received the nuptial blessing, Basilio "started nimbly to his feet and with unparalleled effrontery pulled out the rapier", going off with his new bride.

Clearly, the second *Don Quixote* has left the sphere of real suicides like Chrysostome's in the first novel (chapter 12), for the sphere of theatre.

Work

Metaphors can be enacted on the stage, and strategies of desire can fight duels without forcing the knight to endanger his life. But he has in no way given up monopolising the conversation. To prevent another fight, "he brandished [his lance] so stoutly and dexterously that he overawed all who did not know him", and delivered a speech on "love and war [that] are the same thing and … make use of wiles and stratagems to overcome the enemy" (De Cervantes, 1605/1615, p. 521).

A confirmed bachelor—"I myself am not married, nor, so far, has it entered my thoughts to be so"—Don Quixote develops at length the antithesis of his original thesis. Love, although necessary for marriage, is not enough. Basilio must abandon his Bohemian lifestyle and engage in lucrative work, lest his wife be assailed by "the royal eagles and birds of towering flight …, ravens and kites and other birds of prey" that attack the fair woman left in "want and penury" (De Cervantes, 1605/1615, p. 523).

His discourse provides food for thought: "it was the opinion of a certain sage … that there was not more than one good woman in the world; and … each one should think that [she] was his own wife" (De Cervantes, 1605/1615, pp. 523–524).

Indeed, Don Quixote eliminates the dichotomy between the virtuous poor man and the villainous rich man. Planted in the ground, his lance restores the *relief* flattened out by right-thinking slogans. It is up to the reader to join the knight in his campaign against imbecility.

After breathing new life into the young, he now sets off to confront a more daunting opponent, in the political arena. Bur first, like warriors of ancient times, he must perform an animist ritual to give himself courage. "One could almost say that man is a ceremonial animal […], something in us speaks […] in favour of those savages", Wittgenstein was to confirm later (1967). (Indeed, these primitive practices continue to exert a profound attraction.)

Cervantes is convinced of it. The go-between who will facilitate Don Quixote's shamanistic journey is none other than Basilio's cousin, a polygraph presenting himself as a humanist, "making books for the press, all of great utility and no less entertainment to the nation". The profitable trade of useless knowledge has always entertained the nation, preventing it from thinking.

Like Avellaneda, the cousin makes use of masterpieces to produce cheap imitations. His next book, which bears the pretentious title *Metamorphoses* or *The Spanish Ovid*, "imitating Ovid in burlesque style", will have no trouble finding a publisher, any more than the cousin's other book, "which treats of the invention of things" and is entitled *The Supplement to Polydore Virgil* (De Cervantes, 1605/1615, p. 525). Sancho throws in his two cents' worth: "can you tell me ... who was the first man that scratched his head? For my thinking it must have been our father Adam. But now tell me who was the first tumbler in the world? [It] was Lucifer."

Responding to his master's surprise at his erudition, Sancho comments: "Nay! To ask foolish things and answer nonsense I needn't go looking for help from my neighbors" (De Cervantes, 1605/1615, p. 526).

Indeed, initiation into nonsense is not a new thing. It is clear that even in Cervantes' time, there were those "who weary themselves out in learning and providing things that, after they are known and proved, are not worth a farthing to the understanding or memory" (De Cervantes, 1605/1615, p. 526). In contrast, memories triggered by the imminent descent into the cave of Montesinos have a very different symbolic charge. Don Quixote asks Basilio's cousin to take him to this mythical place.

Nekuia: visiting the land of the dead

The cave, whose exact location is known, is still unspoiled and can be visited as long as one carries a flashlight. Like Ulysses, Aeneas, and other heroes, Don Quixote prepares to undertake a veritable *nekuia* through one of those crevices in the earth the Celts in Ireland called St Patrick's Purgatory (Le Goff, 1986).

The cave's entrance, hidden by green alders, is guarded by birds of ill omen: crows, owls, and bats that come to collide with the knight's face. It is two o'clock in the afternoon. The time is noted with precision, for in the world of surviving images we are about to enter, the course of time has been altered.

On the threshold of the ceremonial space, it is crucial to rope up to confront the Beyond.

"Tie me and hold thy peace" are the last words that Sancho hears.

After that, Don Quixote crosses over to the other side of the visible world, entrusting himself to his Lady, "to precipitate, to sink, to plunge ... into the abyss before [him], only to let the world know that while thou dost favor me there is no impossibility I will not attempt to accomplish" (De Cervantes, 1605/1615, p. 527).

The action unfolds like in a silent movie, accelerating the motion to show the urgency of retrieving lost time. Don Quixote's voice is no longer heard. The rope is let down into the depths of the "dread cavern", then pulled up slowly, with no weight at the end of it, until, after a half hour of suspense and worry, a weight is felt on it again. Brought back into the light of day, the hero plunges into deep sleep from which he has trouble awakening. Contrary to the hell of the fulling hammers (De Cervantes, 1605/1615, p. 117) in the first novel, this "beyond" is not in the least dreadful: "God forgive you, friends; ye have taken me away from the sweetest and most delightful existence and spectacle that ever human being enjoyed or beheld."

It is time for a debriefing. Following the example of Cardenio, the madman of the Sierra Morena, they adopted a reclining position, favourable for conducting an Antiquity style symposium: "all three sitting down [on the grass] lovingly and sociably, they made a luncheon and a supper of it all in one". Once the picnic cloth was removed, Don Quixote addressed his companions in a solemn tone: "Let no one rise, and attend to me, my sons, both of you" (De Cervantes, 1605/1615, p. 528).

It is four in the afternoon. The speleological expedition took one hour at most, but for the hero, in a mystical dimension, it lasted three days and three nights, without sleep or nourishment—which explains his great hunger. The story he is about to tell is a slightly modified version of the catharsis which occurred at the Lake of Boiling Pitch.

After stopping to rest on a ledge of the cave wall, he was plunged into a trance-like sleep; when he awoke, he wondered if he was still himself and "whether it was I myself who was there or some empty delusive phantom" (De Cervantes, 1605/1615, p. 528). In this other world, he recognises the "delightful meadow [and] stately castle, with walls that seemed built of clear transparent crystal", an exact replica of Teresa of Avila's "interior castle" of the soul. But this time, when the castle doors open, instead of beautiful young maidens, the knight sees "a venerable old man" advancing towards him. Montesinos himself, with his snow-white beard, the hero after whom the cave is named, tells Don Quixote his story.

After the promise made to his brother in arms Durandarte, killed at the battle of Roncesvalles, to take his heart to Lady Belerma, the reader is given all the details regarding the extraction and cleaning of the heart, including the sprinkling of salt "to keep it sweet" (De Cervantes, 1605/1615, p. 529).

The theme of a shared heart is a traditional one in courtly love (Neilli, 1974, p. 90). Indeed, seven hundred years or so have passed, with time standing still in a sphere where all the living dead enchanted by "Merlin, who they say, was the devil's son" (De Cervantes, 1605/1615, p. 530), are waiting for the knight to deliver them. These were "the marvels hidden within this transparent castle".

Don Quixote has just undertaken a "vision quest", as the Lakota Indians of South Dakota call it, with only one difference. To seek their vision, the Sioux Indians climb to the top of a hill, wrapped naked in a star blanket. In contrast, the knight descended into the depths, fully dressed. But, upon his return, he recounted what he saw, just as they do.

The mouth of the cave is located on the cliffs overlooking the magnificent green Lagoons of Ruidera, which are fed by the Guadiana River. Don Quixote saw with his own eyes the lagoons regain their original human form. Duena Ruidera, her seven daughters, and two nieces were "changed into so many lakes [by] Merlin, because of the tears they shed", while the squire-river Guadiana, greatly grieved at having to leave Montesinos, "plunged into the bowels of the earth, [whence] he from time to time comes forth.... The lakes aforesaid send him their waters, and with these, and others that come to him, he makes a grand and impressive entrance into Portugal" (De Cervantes, 1605/1615, p. 532).

The message is clear and simple. The knight's mission is to lift the enchantment. The one most concerned, with his embalmed heart, does not set such great store by Don Quixote's powers as a shaman. "And if that may not be, said the wretched Durandarte in a low and feeble voice, ... then, my cousin, I say 'patience and shuffle'" (De Cervantes, 1605/1615, p. 532).

Here, Cervantes the poet lends his voice to the resurgences of time and to the animist practices seen in the Spanish countryside he criss-crossed for twenty years, after his return from the bagnios in Algiers. Drawing inspiration for his *Galatea* from Ovid's *Metamorphoses,* he turns Don Quixote into a seer. After Montesinos has spoken, the knight heard "a great outcry and lamentation, accompanied by deep sighs and bitter sobs, [and saw] a procession of two lines of fair damsels all clad in mourning", followed by the famed duena. After this, Cervantes seems to have developed a taste for musicals.

When Lady Belerma enters the novel, she embodies a bygone era as well. This aging Dulcinea is as old as the knight and resembles Villon's Belle Heaulmière (1489b, p. 124): "her nose was rather flat, her mouth was large but with ruddy lips, and her teeth … were seen to be sparse and ill-set, though as white as peeled almonds. [She had] great dark circles round her eyes, and [a] sickly complexion … not caused by the periodical ailment usual with women, for it is many months and even years since she has had any" (De Cervantes, 1605/1615, pp. 532–533). She carries in her hands the mummified heart of her lover Durandarte, who, mummified or not, did not hesitate to shuffle the cards.

At this point, Montesinos makes the blunder of comparing Belerma to Dulcinea. "Hold hard!" interjects Don Quixote, adding "you know very well that all comparisons are odious".

Nevertheless, introducing this Lady of a certain age serves to taunt the forger who made fun of Cervantes' age. Sancho was surprised that upon hearing this sacrilegious comparison, his master did not assault his host: "I wonder that your worship did not get upon the old fellow and bruise every bone of him with kicks, and pluck his beard until you didn't leave a hair in it" (De Cervantes, 1605/1615, p. 533).

Instead, Don Quixote has gained new energy in the land of the phantoms of History, to which he has become an eye-witness.

"Primitive animism"

> I saw with my own eyes [they] neither eat, nor are they subject to the greater excrements.
>
> (De Cervantes, 1605/1615, p. 534)

"But where are the snows of yesterday?" (Villon, 1489a). When literature falls under the auspices of marketing, the Lady finds herself bankrupt. Sancho himself has contributed to this psychological bankruptcy by inventing a vulgar Dulcinea. Don Quixote spotted her in the cave, and was distressed to see her condescend to beg him for a handout.

While protesting that he is no Fugger—the Rothschild of that era, a German banker from Augsburg—he gives the lady's envoy four *reales*. Instead of making a curtsy, the damsel cuts a caper, "springing two full yards into the air". To Sancho's great surprise, he understands that Don Quixote was not taken in by his tricks when, at the end of his narration, his master tells him: "not being experienced in the things of the world, everything that has some difficulty about it seems to thee impossible" (De Cervantes, 1605/1615, p. 536).

He might have said the same thing to his disciple, Sigmund Freud, who attributed the phenomena of the uncanny to "primitive animism" (Freud, 1919, p. 219), advising him to resort to the "association of practices" advocated by Wittgenstein (1967). At the "crossroads of dreams"—where Noh theatre places such visions—the truth of emerging forms, as Don Quixote insists, "admits of neither reply nor question".

The rationalist Cide Hamete is as sceptical as Freud. Hamete recorded his doubts on the margin of the manuscript: "I cannot convince or persuade myself that everything that is written in the preceding chapter could have precisely happened to the valiant Don Quixote: ... he [who] would not have told a lie though he were shot to death with arrows" (De Cervantes, 1605/1615, p. 537).

How can we resolve the contradictions of this aporia? Once again, the reader is asked to distinguish between fraud, fiction, and historical truth: "Decide for thyself in thy wisdom, reader." If the reader is well versed in literature, he can refer to Plato's "Myth of the Cave", in which the projected shadows are surviving forms of ideas (*eideia*) glimpsed by the psyche before its fall. If the reader has no ideas, instead of braying like a donkey, as Sancho would do shortly, he had best turn to stories and songs which, like *Don Quixote*, are within everyone's reach.

In fact, in the end Don Quixote admits that he invented the episode about the cave in order to punctuate his new adventures with a visit to local divinities (De Cervantes, 1605/1615, p. 767). For Cervantes is now directing the heroes towards a ducal palace which, behind a cultured and refined appearance, will gradually be shown to be just as brutal and stupid as the kingdom of *Ubu Roi* (King Ubu) (Jarry, 1896).

They say I am off to war

Don Quixote's expedition continues to follow closely upon the early traces of young Cervantes' journeys. Now, the knight crosses the path of a man on foot, leading a mule loaded with lances and halberds, followed by a youth who "might have been eighteen or nineteen; … and he went along singing *sequidillas* to beguile the wearisomeness of the road" (De Cervantes, 1605/1615, p. 539). At the age when he left for Italy, Cervantes might have sung, like the youth: "I'm off to the wars/ For the want of pence, /Oh, had I but money/I'd show more sense."

When we were children, we used to sing a Piemontese song about the soldier whose beloved refuses to grant him a kiss:

> Why should I let you kiss me
> When they all speak ill of thee,
> They say you are off to war,
> In the Piedmont, to serve his majesty.

The lover confirms these rumours, making a promise worthy of a Dulcinea:

> I shall love you my whole life through,
> And love you still from the beyond,
> If this be granted to the dead, the dead and gone.
> (De Cervantes, 1605/1615, p. 540)

Like in the song, the young man "would rather have the King for a master, and serve him in wars, than serve as a court pauper". Don Quixote reiterates his discourse on Arms and Letters, to prepare him for the fate that might await him, be it stepping on a mine or being killed by a cannonball. He delivers a lesson in stoicism:

> Remember, my son, that it is better for the soldier to smell of gunpowder than of civet, and that if old age should come upon you in this honorable calling, though you may be covered with wounds and crippled and lame, it will not come upon you without honor, and that such as poverty cannot lessen.
> (De Cervantes, 1605/1615, p. 541)

The new recruit makes it possible for the old soldier Cervantes to transmit a message that is still timely concerning the need for granting pensions to discharged soldiers, and particularly to those bearing physical or psychic wounds, whose traumas ceaselessly resurface, well into their old age.

The reader suspects, of course, that the war traumas analysed in the first novel are ready to re-emerge in the second. He can foresee that the inn where the heroes are about to arrive will be the preferred site where such resurgences occur. When they reached it, "it was not without satisfaction that Sancho perceived his master took it for a real inn, and not for a castle as usual" (De Cervantes, 1605/1615, p. 541).

Indeed, Don Quixote displays his sense of reality by helping the man with the halberds to take care of his beast, with "a degree of humility which made the other feel bound to tell him" (De Cervantes, 1605/1615, p. 542) the purpose for which these arms were intended.

Making an ass of oneself

The story of the halberds starts with the search for a lost ass, found devoured by wolves, like the carcass of Cardenio's mule in the First Part of the novel. To find the animal, two village *regidors* agree to bray in the forest, so that the ass might answer them. The two grandees end up forgetting the objective of their mission, and exchange endless compliments regarding their powerful "organs". Their exchange takes the tone of the *Donkey's Mass*, celebrated in the Notre Dame Cathedral in Paris, during the Feast of the Innocents, between Christmas and New Year: "And I say too that there are gifts going to loss in the world", exclaimed one of the brayers. To which the other replied: "if the abbot sings well, the acolyte is not much behind him" (De Cervantes, 1605/1615, p. 544).

The Feast of Fools is in full swing when "the devil, who never sleeps", causes everyone to start braying, literally and figuratively, sounding the bugle call for an imminent war which draws in the whole population. In Rabelais' version (c. 1532–1564), the jester Panurge throws a sheep into the sea, the others soon jump in after it to follow their bleating leader, and the sheep vendor jumps in with them. A breath of madness is astir in inflamed minds: "Then the boys took to it, which was the same thing for it as getting into the hands and mouths of all the devils of hell; and braying spread from one town to another …, and neither king nor shame, can mend matters" (De Cervantes, 1605/1615, p. 544).

This time, the theatre of war is the land of peasants, ravaged by civil wars and wars of religion. Don Quixote's third sally takes place in a Spain in which the Moors, after the Jews, were chased out of Spain due to the fanatical jackasses of the Inquisition.

Duly informed by the man with the halberds of what is happening in the region, Don Quixote joins the guests at the inn, where he will witness the return of a disquieting character.

Monkey business

Master Pedro, alias Gines de Pasamonte, makes a comeback in the second novel, with a divining ape. He is preceded by his reputation as a seer and puppet showman, but we glimpse a scoundrel under the patch covering half his face. His divining ape whispers in his ear, delivering a prognosis of things past and making him very rich in the process. His skills fascinate the innkeeper, but Sancho is not impressed: "Gad, I would not give a farthing to be told that what's past with me, for who knows that better than I do myself?" (De Cervantes, 1605/1615, p. 545).

Don Quixote is not taken in either. He distrusts the monkey business of the master ape tamer, because his seismograph has detected trickery in the showman's performance. The knight has seen this before. After suspecting that Pedro "has a pact, tacit or express, with the devil" (De Cervantes, 1605/1615, p. 547), he smells one of those quacks who "bring to naught the marvelous truth of science by their lies and ignorance" (De Cervantes, 1605/1615, p. 547).

Like all of us, "Don Quixote was thunderstruck"; he was astounded, at least consciously, and took the bait, while madness set its lie detector to work. Certain predictions derided by medieval sotties (Aubailly, 1984) still foretell a hopeless future for so-called mental illness, augmenting the fortunes of modern apothecaries by bringing to naught, through their ignorance and greed, the marvellous truth of scientific biology.

Small wax candles are lit around the stage on which the puppets handled by Master Peter will enact "the release by Senor Don Gaiferos of his wife Melisendra, when captive in Spain at the hands of the Moors". Based on the Spanish *romanceros* of the Middle Ages, the story narrated by a young boy suddenly propels the knight into action. He rushes to Melisendra's rescue, just as he did to save Queen Madasima when Cardenio spoke ill of her (De Cervantes, 1605/1615, p. 159). The entire episode was set to music in 1923 by Manuel de Falla, in his opera *Master Peter's Puppet Show* (Canavaggio, 2005, pp. 192–193).

This time, the reader understands that the danger is right on the Lady's doorstep, which is to say, on Cervantes' doorstep. Indeed, Melisendra was made captive in Saragossa, the very place where the counterfeiter carried out his forgery. As Don Quixote has demonstrated ever since his encounter with the Knight of the Mirrors, there is no use trying to talk with a pervert. So he ends up smashing Master Pedro's face, as it were, by ruining his puppet show.

No sooner said than done. He jumps on the stage, attacks the hostage-takers, and destroys the miniature castle, not without setting right an error in the historical content of the plot: "bells are not in use among the Moors, only kettledrums". Don Quixote sees Master Pedro's indifference to detail as an indication of his deep-rooted dishonesty. The contempt shown for his ideals causes him to go completely berserk, and at the same time avenge the outrage against his father: "Never, while I live, will I permit foul play to be practiced in my presence on such a famous knight" (De Cervantes, 1605/1615, p. 552).

The reader, who remembers what message he was told to deliver to the counterfeiter, has no trouble recognising Cervantes in the puppet character Don Gaiferos who carries off his Lady, rescuing her from the Moors following them in hot pursuit:

> Suiting the action to the word, he drew his sword, and with on bound placed himself close to the show, and with unexampled rapidity and fury began to shower down blows on the puppet troop of Moors, knocking over some, decapitating others ..., and at length, in less than the space of two credos, he brought the whole show to the ground, with all the fittings and figures shivered and knocked to pieces.
>
> (De Cervantes, 1605/1615, p. 552)

A word to the wise! The swindler's laments reveal his mercantile conception of artistic creation: "And whose were the bodies they belonged to but mine? And what did I get my living by but by them?" (De Cervantes, 1605/1615, p. 553).

The allusion to the pimp's business is explicit. Don Quixote, whose father was also treated like merchandise, admits that he had taken words for things, as happens when words lose their consistency: "I assure you that to me everything ... seemed to take place literally." Therefore, he is willing to compensate Master Pedro fairly: "Let him have [what he wants], Sancho, not to catch the ape (which has escaped in the confusion)—but to get drunk" (De Cervantes, 1605/1615, p. 554).

The first round of the Cervantian vendetta, with an acting out worthy of the first novel, culminates in a good meal, when "all supped in peace and good fellowship at Don Quixote's expense, for he was the height of generosity" (De Cervantes, 1605/1615, pp. 554–555). But the Arab chronicler Cide Hamete has some unanswered questions regarding Don Quixote's fit of madness. He therefore reminds the reader of Master Pedro's true identity: Gines de Pasamonte in the First Part of the book. Hemete's enquiries reveal that his latest swindle consisted of "[informing] himself at the nearest village" before giving a show, to impress the gapers with his "divining" ape. "In this way he acquired a prodigious name and all ran after him" (De Cervantes, 1605/1615, p. 557).

This brings to mind all those who pretend to see the invisible scenes in the *Marvellous Puppet Show*. In this *entremes*, the most famous of Cervantes' interludes, revived in the 1930s by Jacques Prévert, Jean-Louis Barrault, and Federico Garcia Lorca, a swindler named Chanfalla shows the audience a white sheet, saying: "no one who has a drop of Jewish blood, or who has not been born of parents locked in legitimate matrimony … shall be able to see, or hear, the wonders of my show" (De Cervantes, 1615).

Although Don Quixote has been warned by his father about the pitfalls of mass psychology, he cannot stop himself from becoming involved in the civil war foretold.

Peace process

When Don Quixote leaves the inn the next morning at eight o'clock to travel to Saragossa, from the top of a hill he sees bands of armed men, as he had once seen herds of sheep; but now, he is not hallucinating. The war of brayers is in full swing. Drums and trumpets accompany this battle, whose ludicrous cause is known to the reader.

Seeing this, Don Quixote "advanced with an easy bearing and demeanor", intending to act as peace negotiator. His speech, which would do honour to a political science graduate, elucidates the concept of legitimate defence as it applies to duels and just war. But, as usual, things go wrong in the passage from theory to practice.

When Sancho wants to tell the crowd, in his own words, about his expertise in the art of braying, he is hit hard with a staff for having mocked a soldier of this holy war. At once, the scapegoating mechanism "crossbows and muskets unnumbered … leveled at the knight";

"[he] took to flight and, without a thought of Sancho or the danger in which he was leaving him, retreated to such a distance as he thought made him safe" (De Cervantes, 1605/1615, p. 561). Obviously, Don Quixote does not measure up to leaders with demagogic arguments.

In this situation of mass frenzy, where the knight's celebrated bravery is sorely tested, the ass drops the squire at Rocinante's feet, "sore, bruised and belabored". Of course, the betrayal associated with the blanketing incident is brought up again (De Cervantes, 1605/1615, p. 562). Once more, the debriefing takes place in a wood serving as a retreat, like so many times before. Don Quixote goes to great lengths to explain the wisdom of retreating in the face of overwhelming odds, but Sancho keeps pointing out his shameful abandon: "every day I am discovering more and more how little I have to hope from keeping company with your worship" (De Cervantes, 1605/1615, p. 562).

Not knowing what to say, Don Quixote evades the question, making reference to the staff blows to explain Sancho's pain. The squire replies sardonically: "By God, your worship has relieved me of a great doubt."

We are seeing "forward psychiatry" at work. In these combat situations, causal reasoning does not apply. Like they did when they conducted their previous sallies, the two heroes engage in a form of exchange which is that of war psychotherapy. Instead of offering him some anger-calming drug, the knight encourages Sancho to speak in the transference against him: "Talk away, my son, say whatever comes into your head or mouth, for so long as you feel no pain, the irritation your impertinences give me will be a pleasure to me" (De Cervantes, 1605/1615, p. 562). And he adds that he is ready to let him return to his village, with everything he has earned paid up: "You have money of mine; see how long it is since we left our village this third time, … and pay yourself out of your own hand."

Sancho seizes upon the occasion to re-open a tough discussion on the wages to which he feels entitled. This time, he inflates the duration of his services from two months to twenty years. Having started with the "thou" of polite conversation, the haggling ends with the use of the casual "you" when, tired of seeing the stakes rise, Don Quixote leaves the negotiating table abruptly. His economic perspective does not reckon in terms of more or less, but on all or nothing, which translates into straightforward sharp insults. He calls Sancho a "perverter of the squirely rules of knight-errantry, … scoundrel, rogue, monster".

The tension rises until the monologue resembles that of Don Diego in Corneille's El Cid:

> O bread thanklessly received!
> O promises ill-bestowed! O man more beast than human being! ...
> Ass thou art, ass thou wilt be, and ass thou wilt end when the course of thy life is run.
>
> (De Cervantes, 1605/1615, p. 564)

Sancho instantly retreats from the class conflict upon encountering the unabashed paternalism of his master, to re-enlist in errantry and re-enter the "space of the marvel"—a term for the forest in the Middle Ages. After resting among the oaks of Toboso and the green cork oaks of their meeting place with Carrasco, they now take refuge in a grove of elms and beech trees, before pursuing their journey and reaching the banks of the Ebro two days later.

"A small boat without oars or any other gear", set in place at the start of the book, when this third sally was planned, is "calling and inviting [Don Quixote] to enter it" (De Cervantes, 1605/1615, p. 565).

Who will take me to the other bank?

Sung over and over, this French canon seems to go round endlessly. Determined to embark no matter what, Don Quixote did not hear his squire's reasonable remarks: "the boat ... belongs to some of the fishermen of the river, for they catch the best chad in the world here" (De Cervantes, 1605/1615, p. 556).

Don Quixote payed no heed, tied their beasts to a tree, "[embarked] and cut the moorings by which the boat [was] held, and the boat began to drift away slowly from the bank" (De Cervantes, 1605/1615, p. 566). In vain did Dapple bray, Rocinante struggle to get loose, and Sancho lament the dismemberment of their plural body; his master, in the role of a new Christopher Columbus, calls him a "cowardly creature". Setting out on a voyage of discovery with an imaginary astrolabe and Ptolemaic calculations, he sees himself crossing the equatorial line, just like "the Spaniards and those who embark at Cadiz for the East Indies" (De Cervantes, 1605/1615, p. 567).

His father's dream of knowing other lands nearly comes true, by dint of geographic and astronomical references: "lines, parallels, zodiacs, ecliptics, poles, solstices, equinoxes, planets, signs, bearings, the measures of which the celestial and terrestrial spheres are composed" (De Cervantes, 1605/1615, p. 567), and of which Cervantes must have dreamed when contemplating an orrery.

His son crosses the line in his place, and asks Sancho to pass his hand down his thigh to check that all the lice are dead—as it is said that they will be when a vessel passes the equinoctial line—"and not a single one is left". But the test showed that the lice were still there, along with many other germs that were already spreading deathly diseases among American Indians.

Giant mills appear on the horizon again, but this time they are watermills. Don Quixote takes them for a castle. Yet, there has been progress since the first novel, for now he admits that "though they look like mills, they are not so" (De Cervantes, 1605/1615, p. 568). Millers covered with flour, armed with long poles to prevent river boats from being sucked in by the draught of the wheels, create the surrealistic impression of a fortress inhabited by spooky creatures; they upset the boat, throwing Don Quixote and Sancho into the water.

Fortunately, the knight knew how to swim: "lucky it was for Don Quixote that he could swim like a goose, though the weight of his armor carried him twice to the bottom" (De Cervantes, 1605/1615, p. 568). Having been saved from drowning, the knight does not relinquish the idea that he has failed to free the persons supposedly held prisoner in the castle. However, he willingly pays for the fishermen's boat smashed by the wheels of the mill, "with great calmness, just as it nothing had happened him".

The two heroes "returned to their beasts and to their life of beasts" (De Cervantes, 1605/1615, p. 569). By referring back to the episode of the windmills, Cervantes lays bare the failures of his own life. Not only did he fail to prevent the hijacking of his first novel, but he also failed to sail for Mexico, Bolivia, or Guatemala, where he would surely have become a man of means. Had he been able to leave Spain, the theft of his work would not have occurred, but neither would he have created the son born of his misfortunes.

Facing perversion

To find a way out of this impasse, Cervantes places his readers in a boat with no oars or rudder, which carries them far away from the boiling lake of war, towards the swirling rapids of the enlightened world. The moorings are released at the successful conclusion of the third sally, in which Don Quixote wins the first duel he has ever fought, strengthens the ethics of matrimony and education, and has a shamanic vision to boot. But after this, the author will plunge him into a period of voluntary servitude, unfolding for two hundred pages and eighteen chapters (De Cervantes, 1605/1615, chapter XXX to chapter XLVII), in the household of a generous, cultivated, and charming couple.

This time, the dream reflects reality. And there's the catch. Now that, at long last, the two heroes are believed, understood, celebrated, supported, and talked about, one would think they would be glad to boast of having gained a place among those in power. What more could they ask for? Cervantes can be proud of his son's success. Perhaps he himself dreamed of becoming a writer at the court or some prince's advisor? As for Sancho, he quickly becomes the darling of the ladies, the favourite protégé of a sponsor, the spokesman for Don Quichote's grand plan, the polisher of his image, his minister of justice, of culture, and of communication.

But the reader, warned in the Preface that he would confront the forger at some point, remains on his guard.

In fact, we are alerted "the next day toward sunset", when the meeting with a graceful huntress introduces the theme of taking prey. This fairy of the forest on a white palfrey, bearing a hawk and riding in the midst of "high-flying" hunters is "splendor itself" (De Cervantes, 1605/1615, p. 570) engaged in high-level predation! Sent to her side by the Knight of the Lions, Sancho is given the same mission the reader was asked to carry out upon meeting the forger. From now on, we must stay alert, for we have come to the heart of the matters discussed in the second novel.

The one who takes herself for Dulcinea

The prey is identified quickly: "a knight so great ..., of whom we have heard a great deal", says the duchess displaying a friendly manner. "Tell me, brother squire, ... this master of yours, is he not one of whom there is a history extant in print?" (De Cervantes, 1605/1615, p. 571).

Overwhelmed with gratitude, Don Quixote is ready to serve her, and she is ready to use him. When the duke enters the scene, the trap closes, creating an institutional setting in which madness feeds the narcissistic satisfaction of the entire team. A plan was drawn up on the spot, and the whole company contrived "to fall in with his humor and agree with everything he said ..., treat him as a knight-errant, with all the ceremonies usual in the books of chivalry they had read, for they themselves were very fond of them" (De Cervantes, 1605/1615, p. 572).

Crash! Bang! It is just at this crucial moment that the heroes give a clumsy performance, Sancho hitching his foot "in one of the ropes of the packsaddle", and his master falling off his badly girthed saddle. The disgrace that accompanies their ceremonial welcome signals the intervention of the unconscious.

In the presence of these lordly figures so confident in their demeanour, they blush, stammer, and stumble, while the duke hastens to show that they are all on equal footing by dismounting from his horse and embracing Don Quixote, who feels "lifted up", basking in a hospitality permeated with second thoughts. Their hosts are delighted "to receive such a knight-errant and such a homely squire in their castle" (De Cervantes, 1605/1615, p. 573), for reasons the reader will be able to decipher, if he is not taken in.

When the duke "went on in advance and instructed all his servants how they were to treat Don Quixote", the hero lost his discernment completely, even that slight doubt that a delusion often keeps alive in secret, to test his interlocutor. He became identified with his character: "this was the first time that he thoroughly felt and believed himself to be a knight-errant in reality and not merely in fancy, now that he saw himself treated in the same way as he had read of such knights being treated in days of yore" (De Cervantes, 1605/1615, p. 574).

The poetry of his delusion is starting to fade. But one of Dulcinea's stand-ins is watching. Proud Dona Rodriguez rejects the false equality of status. "All aglow with anger", she insults Sancho, who is asking her to keep Dapple company, "for the poor little beast ... cannot bear being alone at all". "Son of a bitch, ... garlic-stuffed scoundrel!" shouts this stern lady, "and what is more, to wind up with, he called me old."

Mozart was inspired by this scene when he composed *The Marriage of Figaro*, in which the word *età*—age—punctuates the Susanna–Marcellina duet, while the audience laughs at the indignation of the old woman.

"Duena Rodriguez is me", could comment Cervantes, who feels the burden of age and prepares for her a grandiose scene in which age will display its best attributes to avenge the hero. In the meantime, a disquieting scenario is taking shape surreptitiously, aiming to separate the two inseparable protagonists.

As soon as they arrive at the castle, the knight counsels his squire regarding proper conversation in such a place. But to no avail: "Senor, everyone must mention what he wants wherever he may be" (De Cervantes, 1605/1615, p. 575).

In vain does Don Quixote call the rebellious squire a "new-fledged buffoon and old booby" (De Cervantes, 1605/1615, p. 576). In vain does he try to teach him what to say and not to say and how to say it; Sancho promises him to keep his mouth shut, like Papageno, but, flattered by the attention the duchess bestows on him, he will not hesitate to paint his master in a less than glorious light.

Making his coming out into refined society, Don Quixote is described as "lean, lanky, and long, with cheeks that seemed to kiss each other inside", a filiform figure reminiscent of a Greco painting, and as vulnerable as a shellfish without a shell. Having heard the story of Don Quixote's adventures, ladies in waiting offer to enact the scene of the crossing of the Lake of Boiling Pitch, but the knight flatly refuses their offer, horrified at the prospect of finding himself as naked as a worm, no matter how much he might have dreamed of it: "However, he said they might give the shirt to Sancho, and [shut] himself in with him in a room" (De Cervantes, 1605/1615, p. 576). We can see here how accurately his unconscious senses the upcoming attacks on his modesty.

The portrait of the pale knight stripped almost bare is far from the picture of a superhero. "The scarlet mantle over his shoulders [and] on his head a montera of green satin"; Don Quixote now displays the colours of the fool's costume in which his father found him in the first place. Presented as a "madman" in the falsified story of his adventures, he now actually appears in the dining room of the castle, delivered by his author with his hands tied, as Hannah Arendt would say, to "a secret society in daylight" (1951), whose reigning mistress is the duchess.

The following story, recounted to an analyst in a psychiatric hospital, is a good case in point to illustrate such power games.

CHAPTER THREE

Accomplices

From one castle to another: Christmas at a psychiatric hospital

Sometimes, the castles of Cervantian dukes have strange subsidiaries. It's cold. It's snowing: the dirty, wet snow of Christmas pavements in Paris.

Here, like in a slow-motion film in which old people and madmen engaged in occupational therapy are made to dance to the rhythm of waltzes, the irreality of the scene is not enough to blot out its immeasurable sadness.

We are in a psychiatric hospital. Just before (just after?) Christmas. The faded garlands provide no clue to the exact date. In any case, the garlands have been there at least since last Christmas; the analyst has seen them just where they are for the past twelve months. No one thinks of removing them in the middle of summer, nor of hanging fresh ones when the holidays draw near.

Most nurses are on vacation. The medical director is there as usual, the team of interns and psychologists is somewhat reduced for a few days. The patients don't notice the difference. At most, the absence of five or six patients given permission to visit their families underscores the time outside time for the outcasts of the world who have not gone anywhere. Tonight (or yesterday), no doubt, a colourful Yule log will add a festive touch to the meal and will be enjoyed, hopefully, if the drug treatment still allows the flavours—strong as they are—to be discerned.

When he runs into the analyst on this cold morning, his chief comments: "You should see the new patient brought in the day before yesterday. A difficult diagnosis." A male nurse points him out in the middle of the desolate group, just after morning coffee. Of course, he stands out in the midst of the bluish pyjamas worn by those who are not even authorised to leave the hospital grounds.

A slim, limber man, his deep-set big blue eyes smiling at everyone, his face is bathed in the light of innocence. An overgrown child? No, his deft, precise gestures are those of an adult; and the relations he has established so quickly with those who share his misfortune show open-mindedness without false commiseration.

The analyst approaches him. He is not going to use the usual formula employed with newcomers: "How long have you been here?" Less than a quarter of an hour ago, another new patient had replied coldly, without looking at him: "What about you?" Just to remind him that the question is implicitly always thrown back at him by those who have stepped through the looking glass: "And you, what are you doing here? How long have you been locked up outside of these bars?" This very morning, when the big electric gate opened slowly to reveal the statue of Mercury holding up a tearful patient, his wings and Caduceus in perfect working order, the analyst had to stop his car for a few minutes to allow an old child—at least fifty he thought—to cross, pulling his minuscule wooden car attached to the end of a string. Had there been an annual toy distribution?

The man with the blue gaze stepped forward. He smiled, making it easier for the analyst to ask: "How do you come to be here?"

He doesn't really know. His family, as well as his wife, insisted that he be confined, after a brief consultation with his parents' doctor. "But I don't feel sick in the least!" he jokes, with a wide smile.

Inwardly, the analyst reacts with the classic "Well, they all say that!" There have even been eminent, humanist psychiatrists who converted this innocence into a symptom designated by a beautiful Greek word: *anosognosia*. The patient does not acknowledge his illness. The madman does not admit that he is mad, which is an additional sign of his madness.

In any case, the conversation focuses on the weather, the holiday season, the sad reality of these forlorn souls shut away in the asylum while outside people are preparing for gift-giving and feasts. Then, he shakes everybody's hand and the analyst does the same, without thinking. The conversation went on for at least half an hour. Now, he is engaging with a little group of listeners won over by his kindness. The analyst promises to see him again in a few days, and he agrees politely.

A nurse has been watching the interchange for a little while, from a distance. He leads the analyst to a private office. "So, you met the new patient. What do you think?" The therapist's dubious frown shows that he can't think much at this point. The nurse continues: "In any case, his family stopped him in time. Imagine, for the past few days he has been posting himself in front of department stores to distribute checks to the children attracted by the Christmas display windows. His parents live in a castle, very wealthy people, but still, we end up seeing everything in this work!"

It's true that we see a lot of things, but making a diagnosis is another story. In fact, after over thirty years of hospital and private practice, the analyst has a hard time with diagnoses. Interestingly, so does the medical director. A gruff and generous man, the one who had referred the new patient to him that morning, he showed the same scepticism when he brought his interns together to introduce them to a "problematic" patient. Far from a regular patient presentation intended to educate would-be doctors, or to glorify the knowledgeable master, it was, rather, a conversation with the young doctors and a few team members. After an hour or so, and a firm promise to the patient that they would talk again soon, the chief would turn to his interns: "Well?" he would ask laconically. Textbooks would be quoted: "Infantile psychosis." A shrug. "Paranoid schizophrenia?" A definite "no" signified by a shake of the head and the beard. After five or six diagnoses are proposed, he rises, leaving his audience to their indecision, or perhaps to muse on something more useful than labels.

It must also be said that this same man, when admitting, with the referring nurse, a particularly agitated or delirious patient, would tell the patient, taking up his pen: "Your present condition forces me to prescribe this medication. Of course, from now on we will aim to reduce the dosage." The analyst was able to work some thirty years in a ward headed by such a psychiatrist. He came from Britanny and had the soul of a Breton sailor on a storm-tossed ship, evident in both his qualities and his faults. His name was Edmond Sanquer. He died ten years ago.

El Dorado: of arms, stones, and blood

The holidays are over. The analyst returns to the hospital every week. Today, the blue-eyed man is waiting for him in front of an office that a nurse has indicated. He has changed clothes. They shake hands. They sit down facing each other.

They take the time to exchange New Year greetings; despite not being short-sighted, it is only now that the analyst finally notices what is written in large burgundy letters, almost half an inch high, across the man's sweater: ACCOMPLICES. "What is this?" It's nothing, just the name of the brand, very famous, very visible. It seems that today those who wear these clothes have been turned into sandwichmen or -women.

Perhaps. Be that as it may, we have now been led out of the asylum through a peculiar exit. It is too early to ask the wearer of the message more questions. But the query has been put forth and the analyst will not let go of it. It is interesting to note the place and function of such messages: they are not subliminal, but spelled out in large letters, even on huge posters, in the middle of a conversation.

So much so that they become part of the landscape, or of the clothes—one doesn't see them. In fact, they are the ones looking at you. The reader will object: the design of a T-shirt is none of a psychoanalyst's business! Still, the analyst cautiously steers the conversation back to the information he learned from the nurse. A big smile.

During the Christmas season, the young man was unable to bear the thought that so many children would have nothing in their stockings, that they had no lit-up Christmas tree, no garlands, no candles. He has read *The Little Match Girl*—the Andersen story that made Bion and his sister scream with fear and anger when their father would read it to them at bedtime (1982, p. 26).

So, this year, he decided to give. He himself is not poor, nor really rich. He has a good job—he is an engineer, has a wife and a little boy. He could not resist his impulse: this Christmas season, he had to give. He thought of the entrances of department stores, where many children gathered, but could only take away mental images of treats and toys, at once displayed and out of reach behind the store windows. So he started to give away cheques all around, to surprised children, some of them pulled away by parents fearing some shady scheme. The cheques were not for large amounts, but enough for sweets and toys to celebrate the season.

He was able to do this for several days. Until he told his wife what he was doing. No doubt frightened, she let his parents know and they took him to the family doctor. So that was the story, he concluded, happy and contrite at the same time.

The analyst did not know what to think. Was this asocial behaviour, or overly social? Was it legal or illegal? But behind his hesitation, there was secret approval of these public offerings. On the spur of the moment, he asked if there was a tradition of giving to charities in the family. This was met with a burst of laughter. Careful: the ACCOMPLICES sign is starting to flash, all its neon lights ablaze. Of course, the analyst cannot read them yet, cannot decipher them letter by letter: he does not know the story. Or perhaps History?

Feeling confident, the young man says that he will tell him the family saga. And, with no stops along the way, they travel together to a time well before the middle of the nineteenth century. That day, they journey for over an hour.

It is the story of a well-to-do bourgeois family, involved in business and finance. Soon, they would also take up politics, at the highest levels. Indeed, it has not escaped the analyst's attention that the patient's family name can be found in history books. One of the young man's ancestors—but not in a direct line, he adds matter-of-factly—has earned a special place in the family story. Again, does this mean History?

South America is already the site of multiple revolutions. Who were the go-betweens who connected the man's ancestor with one of the rebel factions? No one knows. Arms must be provided, a large quantity of arms, perhaps for a good cause ... In any case, the transaction that ensued was very profitable and is still very profitable today. Very.

The analyst asks if this kind of illegal trade was in accord with the official position of the ancestor. Again, a burst of laughter: "You know, one can always make arrangements to get around the law. I have even heard some of my uncles say that laws are made to be broken. There are men who take care of these things; in fact, they are called lawmen."

Now the story reveals a darker side and becomes harder to understand for the analyst, who is not a lawman. The ancestor fills up a cargo ship; "with the arms he has bought", the therapist ventures; "No, no, you don't get it at all!"

Indeed, the financial expert/businessman/politician has the ship filled with paving stones. The analyst is more and more puzzled: illegal or not, such a story—even one of arms trafficking—must come to some conclusion. Let us continue. The businessman gains the complicity of the captain. While another ship, also an accomplice, is in close proximity, the captain of the first ship blows it up with all its cargo. Sailors were killed, of course, but the story does not say how many. Everything has a price, doesn't it, and you can't make an omelette without breaking eggs, right? Repulsed by these culinary images, the analyst now feels the limits of morality and indignation have been overstepped. He can't really say if the arms trafficking in itself was a criminal offence or a felony, to use legal jargon. But this last event was clearly assassination, a segment in a chain of complicities that surely involved more than two or three petty thieves.

And that's not all, he went on, with genuine sadness. His ancestor had taken out a huge insurance policy to cover the risks of this explosive ship transport. In brief: he kept the cash of the revolutionaries who were later defeated. He bought no arms and he received the money paid out by the insurer. Moreover, he could not be accused of arms trafficking: who could blame him for having sent stones to South America? The financial result was great wealth, perhaps only one part of the source of the family fortune. Complicity is a powerful social link.

"You know", the young man reassures the analyst, who is brooding over possibly dangerous state secrets, "everyone in the family knows this story. Of course, the prescription limit has come into effect by now." "It would be called amnesty today, that is, literally, prohibition from memory." "That's right. In the family, whenever someone wants to talk about it, he is quickly rebuked: 'It's all just gossip spread by scandalmongers. Nothing has ever been proven or brought to trial. It may all be mere delusion'."

The eleven capital letters ACCOMPLICES have stopped flashing. This word has brought the analyst back to the asylum, and to his responsibilities. He addresses the young man, connecting this fraudulent, criminal fortune to his activities of redistribution of the past few days. "In truth, you are trying to redeem the family name, to save it from infamy and dishonour. My own inclination would be to congratulate you." They set an appointment for the following week, at the hospital, or at the clinic if the young man is discharged beforehand.

The analyst goes to see the medical director right away. "In any case, he is not delusional when he redistributes dirty money, not to say blood-stained money. He displays the old crime to the whole world." In a few words, he explains that based on the terms of the law governing psychiatric hospitalisation in France, this young man should not be there.

"You take responsibility for what will happen afterwards?"

Without hesitation, the analyst pledges his word. The patient left the hospital that evening and never came back.

But before folding and putting away the sweater which has now accomplished its mission in the transference, we should try to find out what becomes of these eloquent objects which point out, in very visible letters, what silent cries cannot express.

Strangely, they are forgotten. Time and time again, with other patients, the analyst had tried, no doubt awkwardly, to speak of these beacons again—unforgettable beacons, since they work to extract an event from oblivion. For instance, the ACCOMPLICES sweater simply dissolved once time was set in motion again. One day, much later, the analyst asked the blue-eyed man what had become of the sweater, which he had never worn again when he came to his appointments. "What sweater are you talking about? I really don't see what you mean. You must be thinking of another patient."

The analyst has to pinch himself to make sure he didn't dream the whole thing up.

The hand pointing to catastrophic times

One day, the analyst became curious about something. He asked the young man, who now came from out of town to see him at the clinic every week, to explain his work in nature protection, as he had described his job when they first talked at the hospital. It had been a long time since his clear laughter had resonated in one of their sessions. It was a laugh that could be called "naïve", keeping in mind that this word shares its root with "native": laughter at the wellspring of laughter. Toying with the analyst's curiosity, he drew closer: "Well, I must tell you first that the carpeting in my office is blue and quite thick."

The analyst was uncomfortable: was this a quirk undetected until now, the kind that caused Bion to be diagnosed as psychotic when he did not answer questions asked of him? The young man was clearly enjoying keeping his interlocutor in suspense. "As I was saying, I arrive at my office at about nine o'clock, after taking my son to school. I greet my colleagues, I look at the mail, if there is any, and I dictate some answers. All this takes me twenty minutes at most."

—And after that?
—After that, I lock the door, I lie on the floor, and I sleep.

Happy with the effect he produced, he goes on:

—I come out a little before noon, I join my colleagues in the dining room, I drink my coffee. Then I go back to my office; it's time for another nap.
—What about your mission to protect us from great ecological catastrophes?
—Listen, the truth is that there is no prevention possible. The critical point has been reached long ago. If nothing happens, so much the better. If something does happen, it will be too late. So I sleep quite peacefully on my blue carpet.

The analyst is stunned. He hesitates between thinking that the young engineer shows incredible philosophical wisdom, and suspecting another form of madness, concealed under the prestige of his professional status.

Some time later, however, the analyst almost returned for advice to the medical director to ask him to intervene in this patient's therapy. For the last several sessions, the latter had seemed more and more nervous. He would stand up, pace back and forth, drawing figures in the air to explain theories the analyst had trouble understanding. His agitation became more intense each week; the analyst was overwhelmed. Several times he arrived with a briefcase, and feverishly took out diagrams bearing the inscription CONFIDENTIAL. The analyst felt more and more uneasy just seeing this red stamp, although he had no idea of what these diagrams showed, and to whom. What if the young man took up his position again in front of department stores, to warn the population and distribute his documents? Was he mad, not mad? Once again, the analyst was in doubt.

But his interlocutor was relentless now. His smile had disappeared. The latest sessions had been punctuated by bitter tears—a child's sobs—running down his cheeks. Armed once more with CONFIDENTIAL circles and ellipses, his speech had become incoherent: "The cows, the grass, the babies ..."

The reader is no doubt getting the impression that there was not much more the analyst and his patient could do together in the office of a clinic. But just that week, between two sessions, the Chernobyl disaster erupted in the media. Not only in the media. In fact, despite the idiotic statement of a politician "in charge", the radioactive cloud had crossed the borders of our country. It had contaminated, for many years to come, the pastures, the mushrooms, the cows, and all the rest. After a few weeks, giving babies their milk had to be prohibited. Had the young engineer been a prophet, or at least a visionary?

In any case, at the next session, the analyst spoke first:

> I must admit to you that you took care of me. And how hard you worked! You understood that there is none so deaf as one who will not hear. This week I finally heard your message loud and clear, on the radio, on television, in the papers. But it's not possible for me and my patients to cause such a great catastrophe each time, just to force me to listen.

The young man seemed pleased with the therapist's reaction. He took the time to explain in detail the consequences, in the mid and long term, of this most serious nuclear accident, which explains the present-day increase in the frequency of thyroid cancer in France and everywhere on the trajectory of the radioactive dust. To say nothing of birth defects in babies born to this day, leukaemias, and other terrible tributes paid to the blindness of man. Moreover, no one can predict when this monstrous debt will end; in the meantime, Moloch is feasting on the leftovers of the so-called consumer society. Who is consuming whom?

For several more months, he kept coming to his weekly sessions. Then he and the analyst decided to put an end to their meetings. There are some people like him, on the lookout for catastrophes all over the planet, who try to warn us. Always in vain. Modern-day Cassandras, they do not always die a violent death like the princess, but sometimes find themselves locked up in the madness of an asylum.

The limits of "causal democracy"

Still, a point of logic remains to be clarified. No doubt that physicians and mathematicians who venture into these catastrophic zones of space and time have much to teach us. Unfortunately, despite his desire to know, the analyst is not equipped to understand or use their scientific models. Instead, he must be content to describe, as precisely as possible, what takes place in the interactions and interferences manifest in these particular transferences.

Such outlandish watchmen let you see at once that they know about betrayal, in soul and body. *Intus* and *in cute*. They have been betrayed by their own, as they say. Their own family, parents, ancestors. They just happen to use the arrow of time in a curious way. Perhaps this is why, when their symptoms insist on revealing a disturbing truth, even one that goes back a whole century, they themselves are called traitors. Traitors to the cause, traitors to their social class, traitors to their brothers: "After all we did for you!"

Yet, from the moment of this original betrayal, which in some cases has taken place well before their birth, they find themselves free of the constraints of ordinary conjugation. Often, they use the present tense even when they tell very old stories. Most of the time, they seem to settle into a present that lacks the consistency of our present, a present without past or future.

But sometimes, rarely, chance events and transferential coincidences occur. In this case, perhaps they took the form of a grandmother who lived with the analyst's family from the time he was born. She was always giving away what little she had. Coincidences and interferences are needed for roads travelled years apart and in different spheres to intersect, creating a junction between a patient and an analyst, the latter acquiring the function of analyst only from that point on. When this happens, there sometimes emerges—like a sad siren rising from the depths, or a haggard survivor carried on the "Raft of the Medusa" forgotten in some dusty museum—an event. Not feelings, desires, representations, or words that might once have been repressed. No; rather, an event out of History, naked, with sharp contours, neither softened nor shaded to make it attractive, acceptable, saleable.

The reader has had to be indulgent to follow the unfolding of the process described so far. As long as we are talking about facts eliminated from History, it sounds simple enough, since we refer to past events that actually occurred. Their traces may have been erased, and sometimes even the traces of the erasure. But, just as a cataclysm sometimes uncovers fragments of civilisations buried by other cataclysms, there was something there waiting to be discovered. This sometimes involves a certain risk. Unimaginative minds can even take this to be the cause of madness in those who come too close to the "forbidden band gap" (an energy gap where no electron states can exist and there is total void; to use the expression of a patient, taken from solid-state physics).

But not so fast! We can't speak of a cause any more as of a *causa nostra* founded on universal acceptance of the causality principle. "There can be no effect without a cause", that's true science, sings the choir celebrating, like Pangloss in Voltaire's *Candide*, "the best of all worlds". The rest matters little. Yet here, the poet unwittingly points to a more rewarding path.

The future waits for us around the corner. Who are these seers, more sensitive than ordinary men to imperceptible yet blinding details, better equipped to amplify the smallest vibration thanks to their damned "seismograph"? We might as well admit now that betrayal by one's own has expulsed a subject from the exclusive system of "causal democracy". But, great God, where is he to go now? Fortunately, there are asylums for that.

Coasting along

Knowing this, let us explore the time dimension. It seems logical to locate the origin at some point in the past: this can simplify all sorts of calculations. With the ephemeris tables, we can always find our bearings. But displacing the origin of the world to some future moment that has yet to exist? Not in order to "foresee" events entirely predetermined by their parameters, like the collision of two trains, or the moment when the bathtub of the upstairs neighbour will overflow into the apartment below. Simply put, this ability to search, the possibility of moving the time pointer freely, is the tool required to explore the time of catastrophes. Future catastrophes are announced by the oracular words of locked-up Quixotic knights.

Welcomed to the Spanish castle of a ducal couple (in French, "castles in Spain" is the equivalent of "castles in the air"), Don Quixote announces the end of the Golden Age.

The lout: attack on linking

Of course, the reception is lavish, and marked by a simplicity that always surprises anyone who is the guest of some grandee: the duke seats Don Quixote in the place of honour, as he was seated at the inn in the first novel, but without the presence of "gentlemen to whom arms are an appartenance by birth" (De Cervantes, 1605/1615, p. 284).

A very long story told by Sancho suggests to the reader what he should think of this great show of pomp and circumstance.

A labourer from his village protested politely when an hidalgo wanted to seat him at the head of his table, "until the gentleman, out of patience, putting his hands on his shoulders, compelled him by force to sit down, saying, 'Sit down, you stupid lout, for wherever I sit will be the head to you'" (De Cervantes, 1605/1615, p. 579).

Sancho is quite aware that Don Quixote does not belong to their world. Already, the duchess had refused his help in dismounting from her horse. She concealed her disgust at the idea of finding herself in his arms, using as an excuse the unworthiness of "imposing so unnecessary a burden on so great a knight" (De Cervantes, 1605/1615, p. 574). Despite his fear of being taken for a freeloader or for "some impostor or swindler" (De Cervantes, 1605/1615, p. 576), Don Quixote has a vague feeling that the in-house rule is the one Rameau's nephew was to formulate later: "The beggar's pantomime [...] is the pantomime of all human kind", which obliges us to "[kiss] the ass of Madame [the mistress of the house] [...] both literally and figuratively" (Diderot, 1776).

At the ducal court, the parasite in chief is an ecclesiastic, "one of those who rule noblemen's houses; [...] one of those who would have the greatness of great folk measured by their own narrowness of mind" (De Cervantes, 1605/1615, p. 577). He has already blacklisted *Don Quixote,* "telling [the duke] it was foolish to read such fooleries". Seeing his position threatened by the two clowns, angry and indignant, he shouts at the "numbskull" Don Quixote, ordering him to go home (De Cervantes, 1605/1615, pp. 579–580).

Without knowing them, the fundamentalist cleric has joined the camp of Carrasco and his accomplices, the barber and the curate. This is enough to send Don Quixote into a fit of prophetic rage, as evidenced by the fact that "trembling from head to foot", he retorted "in a hurried, agitated voice", driving the cleric away, with no objection from the duke and duchess, who were howling with laughter.

The knight pretends that he is no more offended now than his father had been by the counterfeiter Avellaneda and by Lope de Vega's venomous attacks, when they spread the word that "no [...] poet is as bad as Cervantes, none so foolish as to praise Don Quixote". Both father and son pretend that they forgive the offenders: "I ought not to feel [...] aggrieved at what that good man said to me; [for] women, children and ecclesiastics [...] cannot defend themselves". Nevertheless, he feels the offence, and he comments: "Is nothing more needed than to get a footing, by hook or by crook, in other people's houses to rule over the masters?" (De Cervantes, 1605/1615, p. 581).

His question is also aimed at the author's enemies, who have intruded into his work as they saw fit. Don Quixote pretends to "care not a farthing if clerks who have never entered upon or trod the paths of chivalry should think [him] foolish".

The cleric has cleared out, leaving the field open to another colonisation, even more underhanded, that Bion was to call an "attack on linking" (1967). It starts with an attack on feudal homage vows, to which Sancho makes reference in his pledge of allegiance: "I have leant upon a good master, and [...] please God I shall be just such another; long life to him and long life to me, for neither will he be in any want of empires to rule, or I of islands to govern" (De Cervantes, 1605/1615, p. 582).

Right away, the duke takes the place of an overlord. He promptly offers a pseudo governor position to Sancho, bought like a common football player. Sancho is quick to pledge allegiance to the prestigious club that pays him so well, while his master congratulates him on the bright future awaiting him. Both are unaware of the plot being hatched against them, "but play their parts perfectly", as I was told by a patient whose madness was also a fight against perversion. The plot consists of the successive elimination of three major symbolic relations in the Quixotic epic: the barber-surgeon, Don Quixote's grandfather; Dulcinea, the Lady of his thoughts; and Sancho, his second in combat.

Attack on the barber-surgeon father

The scene opens with a laundering ceremony which reintroduces the barber's basin. Symbolic gadget of Cervantes' father, it is the first pillar of the knight's loyalty. The small step separating diversion from perversion is lightheartedly taken by the servants. Without their masters' knowledge, they have planned to play a mischievous trick so as to gain favour with them at the expense of their guests.

The damsels from whom Don Quixote thought he had gotten away arrive in a procession, the first one carrying that very basin, the second a silver jug, and the third white towels on her shoulders. As for the fourth damsel, she both soaps and soft-soaps the unsuspecting knight. Then, pretending that there is no more rinse water, they leave him exposed to ridicule, "the strangest and most ludicrous figure that could be imagined

[…], with half a yard of neck, and that uncommonly brown, his eyes shut, and his [face] full of soap" (De Cervantes, 1605/1615, p. 584).

What a scene! Right out of some French Sottie. Created in the fifteenth century by the law schools of the Latin Quarter in Paris, these plays enacted mock trials in which the powerful were severely and joyfully basted. But here the situation is quite different. This scene of public humiliation is sponsored by those in power. The young people at the castle make fun of Don Quixote's outdated appearance and his literary fame. Now that he no longer rushes into battle, he becomes the passive target of a mock massacre.

And this is only the beginning. In the background, the reader may be hearing Cervantes' reference to Plato's analysis of the origin of tyranny, in *The Republic*:

> The father grows accustomed to descend to the level of his sons and to fear them […]; the master fears and flatters his scholars […]; young and old are all alike; and the young man is on a level with the old, and is ready to compete with him in word or deed; and old men condescend to the young and are full of pleasantry and gaiety […]. The excess of liberty, whether in States or individuals, seems only to pass into excess of slavery.
>
> (Plato, 380 BC)

Complicit in the scheme, the ducal couple lets their guest be ridiculed by

> the concocters of the joke, [who] kept their eyes down, not daring to look at their master and mistress; and as for them, laughter and anger struggled within them, and they knew not what to do, whether to punish the audacity of the girls, or to reward them for the amusement they had received from seeing Don Quixote in such a plight.
>
> (De Cervantes, 1605/1615, p. 584)

Voyeurism is on the agenda in a "society of the spectacle" (an expression coined by French writer Guy Debord), where the duke attempts to regain control by having himself be shaved in his turn. But he does not have the power to prevent the surge of sadism in the kitchen, where the kitchen boys grabbed Sancho in order to shave him using "water that from its color and impurity was plainly dishwater" (De Cervantes, 1605/1615, p. 589).

Attack on Dulcinea

During this "washing ceremony", the psychological war attacks head on the second pillar of Quixotic wisdom. Questioned publicly about Dulcinea's beauty, he confesses, in all honesty: "a few days back [...], I found her enchanted and changed from [...] fair to foul, from an angel into a devil, from fragrant to pestiferous, from refined to clownish, from a dignified lady into a jumping tomboy" (De Cervantes, 1605/1615, p. 586).

The accomplices of Cervantes' enemies show, in real time, the plot they are hatching against him: "Enchanters have persecuted me, enchanters persecute me still, and enchanters will continue to persecute me until they have sunk me, and my lofty chivalry, in the deep abyss of oblivion" (De Cervantes, 1605/1615, p. 586).

The erasure of traces and soul murder are always practised in tyrannical regimes. But Don Quixote rises to the occasion and makes no pleas that would excite his torturers. He gives them a perfect definition of the Lady, which will simply not lend itself to their materialist perspective. "they injure and wound me where they know I feel it most. For to deprive a knight-errant of his lady is to deprive him of the eyes he sees with, of the sun that gives him light, of the food whereby he lives. [...] a knight-errant without a lady is like a tree without leaves, a building without foundation, or a shadow without the body that causes it" (De Cervantes, 1605/1615, p. 586).

Yet the duchess raises doubts as to the existence of the Lady, revealing her own limitations. Restricted to the sphere of mundane pleasures, her narrow mind has no access to the poetic. She insinuates that "the lady Dulcinea [...] is nothing in the world but an imaginary lady, one that you yourself begot and gave birth to in your brain". Despite her ostentatious self-assurance, she cannot hide her ignorance, and keeps missing the point. Don Quixote tries to elevate the level of the discussion, but in vain. Through him, Cervantes asserts that the Lady is a "surviving image"—as Aby Warburg, a future Don Quixote, would call her—making it possible to survive the ambient idiocy.

> God knows whether there be any Dulcinea or not in the world, or whether she is imaginary or not imaginary; these are things the proof of which must not be pushed to extreme lengths. I have not begotten nor given birth to my lady, though I behold her as she needs must be, a lady who contains in herself all the qualities.
>
> (De Cervantes, 1605/1615, p. 587)

Emerging at the place where words fail, she does not belong to the imaginary order of things reflected in the mirror, since her image is indefinable. She appears in the place of nothingness, when there is nothing left to desire, when everything one believes in has been spoiled, and she creates the possibility of a desire to live which cannot be destroyed, even if, concretely, a murder plot has been hatched: "I am of tender flesh and not at all impenetrable; […] I have already seen myself thrust into a cage. […] But as I delivered myself from that one […], these enchanters […] revenge themselves on what I love most, and seek to rob me of life by maltreating that of Dulcinea" (De Cervantes, 1605/1615, p. 588).

Without knowing it, Don Quixote lists the mistreatments inflicted on his father's writing: "smitten, […] altered, changed, and transformed", and he vows to fight "until I see her in her pristine state". Questioned on the Lady's credentials, Don Quixote answers without missing a beat: "Dulcinea is the daughter of her own works, and […] virtues rectify blood, and […] lowly virtue is more to be regarded and esteemed than exalted vice".

A word to the wise! When the knight assures the duchess that "the merit of a fair and virtuous woman is capable of performing greater miracles; and […] she has in herself higher fortunes" (De Cervantes, 1605/1615, p. 587), his unconscious hits the nail on the head. Indeed, the woman who is questioning him might be beautiful—with artificial help, as we shall learn—and of noble birth—but a high-born lady can be highly vicious, for she does not have a gift for joy, only an addiction to perpetual excitement. As for miracles, she alone thinks she can perform them, by spending huge sums on culture and on the latest celebrities. With her, everything is calculated, and she has trouble understanding Don Quixote when he declares that the Lady is not subject to controls:

> your highness must know that everything or almost everything that happens me transcends the ordinary limits of what happens to other knights-errant, whether it be that it is directed by the inscrutable will of destiny, or by the malice of some jealous enchanter.
>
> (De Cervantes, 1605/1615, p. 587)

The Lady is the touchstone of "worthiness" and, as such, the form she takes does not matter. Dulcinea, like the French fairy Melusine (D'Arras,

2013), can change into a serpent, or into a peasant woman. Without knowing it, Don Quixote has put the duchess in her place.

Attack on the therapon

Now, the duchess attacks the third pillar of the knight's loyalty. She has astutely spotted the chink in the armour of the plural body formed by Don Quixote and Sancho: "I cannot help entertaining a doubt, and having a certain grudge against Sancho Panza." And she makes use of Sancho's story of having visited Dulcinea, who was busy sifting wheat, and about whom he had said: "She is as much enchanted as my father" (De Cervantes, 1605/1615, p. 589).

Don Quixote has been under no illusion regarding his squire, who delights him with his unpredictability: "sometimes there is a simplicity about him so acute that it is an amusement to try and make out whether he is simple or sharp". His cunning is proof of his freedom: "he has mischievous tricks that stamp him rogue, and blundering ways that prove him a booby; he doubts everything and believes everything" (De Cervantes, 1605/1615, p. 588).

In short, the knight realises that the discussion is beginning to sound like a job interview, and puts an end to it by declaring: "After all, I would not exchange him for another squire, though I were given a city to boot."

Yet, because their relation is not one of master and slave—something Cervantes had actually experienced—the knight recommends his squire for the highest of positions: "with a little trimming of his understanding, he would manage any government [...], for there are a hundred round about us that scarcely know how to read, and govern like gyrfalcons".

Although the duke and duchess, for their part, know how to read and write, the management of their household is not quite up to the mark. They have no idea that in the servants' quarter, Sancho is being persecuted by the kitchen boys. When Sancho bursts into the reception room "all glowing with anger, with a straining cloth by way of a bib, and followed by several servants", the sottie continues to unfold. "In a great rage" against these "cirimonies", he demands justice and equality before the law: "there is not so much difference between me and my master". Don Quixote rushes to his defence, agreeing entirely with Sancho's opinion that "ceremonies and soapings of this sort are more like jokes than the polite attentions of one's host".

A lesson in human rights. Cervantes knows that legal action is rarely brought for psychological harassment when buckets of dirty water are poured with the best of intentions, in the intimate sphere of the family circle or among friends, and that rarely does anyone intervene to stop it. The sight of the duchess "ready to die with laughter when she saw Sancho's rage" is not to the knight's liking; but he weighs his words and, instead of delivering punches, puts the servants in their place: "Holloa, gentlemen! You let that youth alone [...]; my squire is as clean as any other person [...]; take my advice and leave him alone, for neither he nor I understand joking"; the sly duchess shows agreement, while continuing to laugh (De Cervantes, 1605/1615, p. 590), setting the tone for the double meaning the reader can easily discern in her speech.

How can one distinguish between catharsis and rhetorical laundering? Throughout the high-jinks planned to ridicule the hero, the ducal couple protects its image by showing good intentions—there is no harm in trying—and condemns the abuses it covertly authorises. Thus, the duchess, indignant, scolds her servants: "you are ill-conditioned and ill-bred, and spiteful as you are, you cannot help showing the grudge you have against the squires of knights-errant".

With her, the advocate of torture chambers enters the stage, holding out a cigarette to the prisoner, to make him let down his guard at the sight of this unexpected good-will. The procedure, well known in the prisons of the Inquisition and the bagnios of the Dey of Algiers, proves effective when applied to Sancho who, feeling he has escaped extreme danger, rushes to kneel before the duchess as if she were his Lady, imploring her to let him "devote [himself] all the days of [his] life" to her service. In exchange, she endeavours to "speak his language", and promises to influence the duke in his favour, intending, in fact, to turn him against his master.

She bids him to meet her, during Don Quixote's midday siesta, "in a very cool chamber, [...] to serve her excellence", and to give her an opportunity to worm secrets out of him. "The history records that Sancho did not sleep that afternoon, but in order to keep his word came, before he had well done dinner, to visit the duchess". Sleep deprivation is a well-known method of increasing vulnerability.

Intelligence service

The brainwashing session takes place in the presence of "all the duchess's damsels and duenas gathered round him, [...] in profound silence".

With a shrug of his shoulders, Sancho consents to sit on an ottoman and the interrogation begins. The interview, which is to be reported to the duke in full, is conducted methodically. First, the squire is to be induced to betray his master by admitting that his visit to Dulcinea, as described in the first novel, was an invention. The alleged offender reveals his conflict of loyalty through his actions: "Sancho [...] got up from his chair, and with noiseless steps, with his body bent and his finger on his lips, went all round the room lifting up the hangings [to make sure] that there is no one [...] listening [...] on the sly" (De Cervantes, 1605/1615, p. 591).

We are reminded of Hamlet about to stab the wall hanging behind which Polonius is hidden (Shakespeare, c. 1599–1602). The squire's unconscious is fully informed that he is under surveillance. Knowingly, Sancho goes along with imitating a staff meeting about a psychotic, where the absent party is denigrated. His master's case can be summed up in three points.

"And the first thing I have got to say is, that for my own part I hold my master Don Quixote to be stark mad, though sometimes he says things that [...] are so wise [...] that Satan himself could not have said them better." Here, we have the so-called humanist diagnosis: "but for all that, really, and beyond all question, it's my firm belief he is cracked". And finally, we come to the test that confirms once and for all the superiority of the caregiver over the patient: "I can venture to make him believe things that have neither head nor tail, like that affair of the answer to the letter, and that other of six or eight days ago, [...] the affair of the enchantment of my lady Dulcinea [...], though there's no more truth in it than over the hills of Ubeda."

His sense of omnipotence makes him forget that Don Quixote was never fooled, since he found the letter in question after Sancho's departure for Toboso. Then, suddenly, the squire stops playing, tired of the game of fools into which he has been drawn. But the harm is done. The first stage of brainwashing leads to the betrayal of one's own, "and his hearers were not a little amused" (De Cervantes, 1605/1615, p. 592).

In the next stage of the proceedings, Sancho himself is suspected of being mad, and therefore incapable of assuming the function he has been promised. "there comes a kind of whisper to my ear", the duchess insinuates:

> A doubt starts up in my mind, [...] that says, "If Don Quixote be mad, [...], and Sancho Panza his squire knows it, and, notwithstanding, serves and follows him, [...] he must be still madder and

> sillier than his master; and that being so, it will be cast in your teeth, senora duchess, if you give the said Sancho an island to govern; for how will he who does not know how to govern himself know how to govern others?"
>
> (De Cervantes, 1605/1615, p. 592)

Hearing this, Sancho might be expected to beg her indulgence. But he is not nearly as vulnerable as she would like, and is, on the contrary, proud of the madness of his loyalty. Relieved—he is finally speaking frankly—he admits that "if I were wise I should have left my master long ago". Sancho has escaped the trap by giving the duchess a taste of her own medicine. A valuable old trick for us to remember!

Busy focusing on the information she thinks she is extracting from him, the duchess is hit instead with a declaration of loyalty: "this was my fate [...]; I can't help it, I must follow him; we're from the same village, I've eaten his bread, I'm fond of him, I'm grateful, he gave me his ass colts, and above all I'm faithful; so it's quite impossible for anything to separate us, except the pickaxe and shovel" (De Cervantes, 1605/1615, p. 592).

The three ass colts are well worth an island to govern, when the evaluation system is based on the value of the given word. Resisting the beguiling promise of recruitment to the rank of governor, Sancho ends up joining the ranks of those who—according to Montaigne's friend La Boéti—"feel the weight of the yoke and cannot restrain themselves from attempting to shake it off [...]. Even if liberty had entirely perished from the earth, such men would invent it. For them slavery has no satisfaction, no matter how well disguised" (La Boétie, 1548). Sancho feels, savours, and imagines himself going as he pleases, in the company of his master, and he thinks twice before serving a lady, no matter how enticingly got up.

Refusing consent

In truth, the only thing Sancho cares about is to save his soul, which the duchess persists in trying to buy. His unexpected turnaround, once he sets aside career advancement, brings to mind the sermon on the mountain: "it may be that Sancho the squire will get to heaven sooner than Sancho the governor. 'They make as good bread here as in France', and 'by night all cats are grey' […]. And […] if your ladyship does not like to give me the island because I'm a fool, like a wise man I will take care to give myself no trouble about it" (De Cervantes, 1605/1615, p. 592). And he goes on to evoke the allegorical Dance of Death painted on church walls, to symbolise that in the world beyond "the prince travels by as narrow a path as the journeyman".

No matter what she thinks, the duchess does not have mastery over life and death. Yet she continues to bully her whipping boy. She uses a classic technique of psychic manipulation consisting of speaking "in his own style", to gain a more intimate understanding of him. Since loyalty is essential to Sancho, she assures him that her loyal husband will not break his promise to make him governor, provided he discloses his political programme. Two short sentences are all he needs to comply: "After having been governor a fortnight, I'll […] know more about it than [about] field labour"; and "with me the good will have support and protection, and the bad neither footing nor access" (De Cervantes, 1605/1615, p. 593).

The duchess finds Sancho's conduct too ethical. So she keeps coming back to his recent lie—Dulcinea's enchantment—to make him feel guilty, while sympathising: "worthy Sancho, though he fancies himself the deceiver, is the one that is deceived". Sancho refuses to be victimised: "as if Sancho was nobody at all, and not the same Sancho Panza that's now going all over the world in books".

However, tired of resisting, he ends up relating everything to her, including his master's visit to the cave of Montesinos. He gives her everything except his soul and his ass, "which, not to mention him by that name, [he is] accustomed to call Dapple" (De Cervantes, 1605/1615, p. 595).

Dapple is Sancho's staunch ally. When the duchess is making an ass of him, he turns the conversation to his donkey, yardstick of a kind of knowledge the lady is obviously lacking. She has not read Apuleius' *The Golden Ass*. But she is no stranger to asinine matters, and the joke is now on her. Worse still, her insistence on using proverbs, like Sancho does, falls flat, and she fails in her attempt to get chummy with him. Thus, he concludes: "I have seen more than two asses go to governments" (De Cervantes, 1605/1615, p. 596).

A word to the wise! Unaware that Sancho's unconscious witticism referred to her, "she went away to tell the duke the conversation she had

had with him, and between them they plotted and arranged to play a joke upon Don Quixote that was to be a rare one and entirely in knight-errantry style". The lavish festival of asinine ducal clowning can begin.

Apocalypse now!

A hunting party is organised in "a wood that lay between two high mountains" (De Cervantes, 1605/1615, p. 597), to hunt for wild boar, but in truth the two heroes are the intended prey. The proceedings—consisting of "occupying various posts, ambushes and paths, and distributing the party in different positions, [so that] the hunt began with great noise, shouting, and hallooing"—are identical to those in use today, except for the weapons, up to the final ritual, when the sacrificed animal is covered with sprigs of rosemary and branches of myrtle.

Neither Sancho nor Don Quixote is caught up in the murderous passion of the duchess, who "dismounted, and with a sharp boar spear in her hand" stood ready to face a huge boar "scattering foam from his mouth; [and she] would have gone in front of them all had not the duke prevented her". The knight advances with the duke to meet the boar, while Sancho—not a fan of hunting except for rabbits and small birds—takes refuge in a tree, breaking the branch and being left hanging upside down. He tears the green hunting coat that he had intended to re-sell as soon as possible. At the foot of the tree, his donkey, less of a brute than the human predators, "did not forsake him in his distress, [...] such was their attachment and loyalty one to the other" (De Cervantes, 1605/1615, p. 598).

Still upset, Sancho criticises "a pleasure which [...] consists in killing an animal that has done no harm whatever" (De Cervantes, 1605/1615, p. 599), while the duke justifies the privilege to hunt big game by presenting it as military preparation. The squire dismisses this argument out of hand: "[These] amusements are more fit for idlers than for governors, [who could have] people coming to look for [them] on business" (De Cervantes, 1605/1615, p. 599).

The idleness of the ruling class, fond of entertainment, is obviously Cervantes' target. At nightfall, a little after twilight in this midsummer season, the traditional hunters' revelry suddenly turns into "warlike" upheaval, not unlike the episode of the *encamisados* (De Cervantes, 1605/1615, p. 111), but even more frightening. "The whole wood [...] seemed to be on fire, [...] a vast number of trumpets and other military instruments were heard, [...] [as well as] repeated lelilies after the fashion of the Moors when they rush to battle" (Schmitt, 1999) in the name of Allah.

Now, a veritable Mesnie Hellequin (De Cervantes, 1605/1615, p. 600) bursts on the scene—the army of Harley, king of the dead, who haunts the forests, filling them with the deafening din of phantoms of young men killed in battle. It was not a good idea, in those times, to linger in the forest at nightfall, as Ronsard found out one evening, when he set out to visit his mistress on the other bank of the Loire. Petrified with fear, as he recounts in "Hymn to Demons" (De Ronsard, 2002, p. 144), he escapes after unsheathing his sword to draw crosses in the air with great determination.

The two heroes are still unaware of the horrific plot mounted against them, thanks to the information provided by Sancho about the cave of Montesinos. Suspense! Hoards of spooky living dead spring into view, more and more terrifying. Terror reigns, making nightmares real and reality nightmarish.

Don Quixote is unmoved, since he has already encountered the ghosts of traumatic revivals in the first novel. Now, a potential space has been opened, allowing him to imagine and reflect on nonsensical scenarios, without becoming confused about their reality. As a result, he does not lose his composure when the devil in person, riding on a chariot, announces the arrival of six troops of enchanters bringing "the peerless Dulcinea [...], together with the gallant Frenchman Montesinos, to give instructions to Don Quixote as to how she [...] may be disenchanted".

The hallucinatory scenes designed to fascinate and terrorise them does not stop the heroes from thinking before they act. Thus, when the fake Devil makes the mistake of swearing "by God and upon my conscience", Sancho notices the slip and tells himself that "there must be good souls even in hell itself", and wonders why "in defiance of the truth, they would have it that Dulcinea was enchanted" (De Cervantes, 1605/1615, p. 601).

His master is just as puzzled, "deep in these cogitations" (De Cervantes, 1605/1615, p. 601), he knows that he invented the visions in the cave of Montesinos. But whatever happens, he is determined to "wait, fearless and firm, though all hell should come to attack [him]". And he will not be disappointed by the performance brimming with special effects: candles, black buckram, penitents, the noise of four battles in the four corners of the woods, hideous demons and old men on four carts in procession, playing enchanters to the sound of music. "where there's music there can't be mischief", says Sancho, feeling reassured, without leaving the duchess's side, taking her for his godmother, as if he were Cherubin and she the Countess in Mozart's *Marriage of Figaro*. "Nor where there are lights and it is bright, she agrees with him" (De Cervantes, 1605/1615, p. 602).

But Sancho is not convinced by those lights, whose false glow resembles the brightness of stakes that "perhaps may burn us", as he puts it; to which Don Quixote replies: "That remains to be seen." And Cervantes adds: "and he was right, as is shown in the following chapter" (De Cervantes, 1605/1615, p. 602).

The allusion to the ordeal of Jews and heretics further intensifies the level of psychological torture.

Psychological harassment

The highlight of this horror play is a cart, three times bigger than the others, on which a veiled nymph is seated on a throne. Beside her, Merlin the Enchanter, in the guise of fleshless and hideous Death, rises to recite a long poem describing the course of action needed to disenchant Dulcinea: "Tis needful that thy esquire Sancho shall, /On his own sturdy buttocks laid to heaven, /Three thousand and three hundred lashes lay" (De Cervantes, 1605/1615, p. 604).

The recourse to torture immediately introduces discord into the relations between the squire and his master. Sancho protests: "I don't see what my backside has got to do with [...] disenchanting the lady Dulcinea del Toboso." Don Quixote threatens to double the number of lashes, adding: "don't answer me a word or I'll tear your soul out" (De Cervantes, 1605/1615, p. 605).

The fake Merlin expands on the exquisite pain of whipping, offering the possibility of reducing the punishment by half, if the lashes are "given by the hand of another, though it may be somewhat weighty". At the height of this ordeal, the nymph uncovers her face, "that seemed to all something more than exceedingly beautiful".

Now, we are at Madame Arthur's transvestite cabaret, where the dazzling beauty "with a masculine freedom from embarrassment and in a voice not very like a lady's", shouts at Sancho, swearing like a sailor: "soul of a pitcher, heart of a cork tree, with bowels of flint and pebbles

[…], impudent thief […], enemy of mankind [with] timorous owl's eyes […], crafty, ill-conditioned monster". The threat of torture escalates when Sancho is made to envision swallowing "a dozen of toads, two of lizards, and three of adders". She brings her monologue to a close with the classic threat to harm his family: "if they wanted thee to slay thy wife and children with a sharp murderous scimitar, it would be no wonder for thee to show thyself stubborn and squeamish" (De Cervantes, 1605/1615, p. 602).

Insults rain down on him in quick succession, in a session intended to exhaust him, such as Cervantes had no doubt undergone in prison and in the bagnios, but which can also be enacted in respectable households and institutions. "Lay on to that hide of thine, thou great untamed brute, rouse up thy lusty vigor that only urges thee to eat and eat" (De Cervantes, 1605/1615, p. 605).

This brings to mind the bullying inflicted on children left in public institutions, who are used to receiving such beatings every month, and to undergoing psychological mistreatment every day. Sancho speaks out, loud and clear, to defend the children who cannot speak up when they are called "a string of foul names that the devil is welcome to". Especially when the adults keep silent and betray them.

But Don Quixote has indeed joined the enemy. He threatens to "tie [Sancho] to a tree naked" and whip him himself if he doesn't comply. Has his loyalty to Dulcinea turned him into a fanatic, as cruel as André's master? (De Cervantes, 1605/1615, p. 25). Or is he seeking revenge for Dulcinea's transformation into a country wench? To top it all off, the duke tries to blackmail Sancho with a veritable Mafioso offer: "unless you become softer than a ripe fig, you shall not get hold of the government".

Using projective identification, he accuses Sancho of the very offences he himself is committing: "It would be a nice thing for me to send my islanders a cruel governor with flinty bowels, who won't yield to the tears of afflicted damsels." Sancho tries to gain time and to negotiate the timing of his self-flagellation, but to no avail. Invoking the excuse that the squire is of "a sanguin habit and it will do [him] no harm to draw a little blood" (De Cervantes, 1605/1615, p. 607). The forerunners of Molière's doctor Diafoirus have a field day in the midst of the general excitement.

Suddenly, with the dawning of a beautiful day, life and poetry regain supremacy. The Green Man and the May Fairy push the horrific visions back into the night. The penitents dressed like members of the Ku Klux Klan leave the stage.

The Green Man

> And now bright smiling dawn came on apace; the flowers of the field, revived, captained up their heads, and the crystal waters of the brooks, murmuring over the grey and white pebbles, hastened to pay their tribute to the expectant rivers; the glad earth, the unclouded sky, the fresh breeze, the clear light, each and all showed that the day that came treading on the skirts of morning would be calm and bright.
>
> (De Cervantes, 1605/1615, p. 608)

In the midst of revival, nature does not give a hoot that the ducal couple prefers to indulge its addiction to games instead of governing its realm "[they] returned to their castle resolved to follow up their joke; for to them there was no reality that could afford [...] more amusement".

As for Cervantes, he seems to say that it's too bad for them if they need sadomasochistic scenarios to awaken their desire. The duchess's repertoire is, in fact, hopelessly repetitive, as we can see by her insistent urging that Sancho should whip himself "with claws, or a cat-o'-nine tails [...] that will be just the thing for you" (De Cervantes, 1605/1615, p. 609).

The phallus of ducal power is obviously firmly lodged in the iron glove of the dominatrix, who interprets literally the Spanish proverb "It's with blood that letters enter", which Kafka illustrated in *The Penal Colony* (1919). In the same way, the duchess requires laceration of "the tenderness of [Sancho's] flesh" (De Cervantes, 1605/1615, p. 609).

Fortunately, the author of the farces she has requested is "a majordomo of a very facetious and sportive turn", who does not feel obliged to be as stupid as his masters. The reader repulsed by raw meat will sympathise. Of course, his instructions are to paint everything black in strict Gothic style—complete with mourning robes, skeletons, and instruments of torture that would terrify anyone except Don Quixote. But the talented steward of cultural events makes the best of the freedom granted by his masters, to produce a breathtaking musical comedy that turns out to work against them.

While he is busy composing it, Sancho attempts to get himself out of the perverse deal which demands that Dulcinea be freed from her spell at the cost of his flesh. To do so, he appeals urgently to his own lady, Teresa Panza. In a letter he dictates for her, he informs her of his promotion: "I mean thee to go in a coach [...]. I send thee here a green hunting suit [...]; alter it so as to make a petticoat and bodice for our daughter."

Then, he summarises his political stance, which places him in a double bind, requiring that he choose between loyalty to his master—"If I am to believe what I hear in these parts, [my master] is a madman of some sense, and a droll blockhead, and I am no way behind him"—and the governor position to which he aspires, "with a mighty great desire to make money, for they tell me all new governors set out with the same desire" (De Cervantes, 1605/1615, p. 610).

Teresa is enjoined to keep secret the "three thousand three hundred lashes" that threaten his backside, for getting a government, Sancho explains, requires consenting to a whipping imposed by higher authorities.

Finally, he tells her that "Dapple [...] sends many remembrances", adding: "I am not going to leave him behind though they took me away to be Grand Turk". He also tells Teresa: "My lady the duchess kisses thy hands a thousand times", which does not cost much—"for [...] nothing costs less [...] than civility"—and the lady must be sent twice that number in return.

The duchess, to whom Sancho showed the letter, disapproves of his covetousness, and wants to remove the reference to whipping, which would paint a poor picture of ducal politics and bring down their score in opinion polls. But Sancho is tired of endeavouring to support his mistress's popularity rating: "if you think the letter doesn't run as it ought to do, it's only to tear it up and make another; and maybe it will be a worse one if it is left to my gumption" (De Cervantes, 1605/1615, p. 611).

The simple act of letting his home front know what is happening to him has given Sancho back the advantage. Disconcerted, the duchess hurries away to show the letter to the duke, and to devise the next plot.

Musical comedy

Now, a music hall show begins, or what was to be called comic opera in future centuries. Music! "A fife and harsh discordant drum" (De Cervantes, 1605/1615, p. 611) produce a doleful sound. The dominant colour is black.

There are four characters in the first act: three musicians in sombre garb, followed by a personage "of gigantic stature", with a long beard as white as snow. His face covered with a black veil, the squire Trifaldin announces the imminent arrival of Countess Doloride, the Distressed Duena, alias Countess Trifaldi or Countess Lobuna, "because wolves bred in great numbers in her country". Here, Cervantes could also be making an allusion to the big bad wolf Lope de Vega, against whom he still holds a grudge. The countess is arriving "on foot and without breaking her fast", to the duke's realm, in quest of the famous gentleman Don Quixote. Since the valiant knight never refuses the protection of his strong arm to any lady in distress, the second act opens with the brilliant ballet of the bearded duenas.

In the meantime, a brief intermission constructed around the signifier Trifaldi—"three-tails"—pokes fun at the duenas' sexuality. Dona Rodriguez defends them in worthy Quixotic fashion, indignant at the harassment inflicted on them by young squires, "our enemies; and [...] the haunting spirits of the antichambers [who] watch us at every step [and] spend their time [...] burying our good name" (De Cervantes, 1605/1615, p. 616). Of course, she is thinking of the disgrace of her own daughter, about whom the reader knows nothing yet.

In fact, her daughter's secret has already been discovered, and is being used by the majordomo in his libretto, featuring the choreographed entrance of a "band of duenas". The melancholy "fife and drums" (De Cervantes, 1605/1615, p. 615) resonate again, followed by twelve duenas advancing slowly in two lines. Behind them, *prima donna* Trifaldi makes her entrance, clad in a black baize dress whose three-point tail is held up by three pages, "likewise dressed in mourning".

The feminine triangle and the three masculine appendages compose "an elegant mathematical figure", who speaks "in a voice hoarse and rough, rather than fine and delicate", that of the transvestite Doloride-Trifaldi. "Kneeling on the ground" before the knight (De Cervantes, 1605/1615, p. 616), she recites her tale of woe in the style "Spoken by Folly in her own person" which opens Erasmus' *The Praise of Folly*: "my strange and unparalleled misfortune has carried off my wits, and I know not whither; but it must be a long way off, for the more I look for them the less I find them" (2010).

A long silence follows, broken at last by a string of sonorous superlatives, like in a Monteverdi opera. The countess speaks of her desire to find the knight "Don Quixote de la Manchissima, and his squirissimus

Panza". The latter, unimpressed with the hyperbole, replies: "La Panza is here, and Don Quixotissimus too, and [...] we are all readissimus to do you any servissimus."

At the apogee of her plea, the countess made as though she would fall at Don Quixote's feet, and actually did, and taking hold of his squire's hands, she asserted that his "goodness is more extensive than the beard of Trifaldin" (De Cervantes, 1605/1615, p. 617).

Sancho seized upon the notion of a beard and used it to create a clever witticism on the leitmotif of Cervantes' barber father: the metamorphosis of Plato's winged souls into bearded souls: "As to my goodness, senora, being as long and as great as your squire's beard, it mattes very little to me; may I have my soul well bearded and moustached when it comes to quit this life" (De Cervantes, 1605/1615, p. 618).

Now, we are told the tale of the troubles of the Princess Antonomasia—a figure of speech that turns a common noun into a proper noun. We learn that the duena was seduced and taken in by pearls of rhetoric. Hearing the tale, the "duke and duchess [...] were ready to burst with laughter [...], and between themselves they commended the clever acting of the Trifaldi" (De Cervantes, 1605/1615, p. 618).

In fact, Antonomasia's fictional story is the real story of Dona Rodriguez's daughter.

The bearded duenas

The maiden in question is fourteen. Born on Taprobane in Hindoustan, an island not far from Ceylon, enchantingly depicted in verse by Luis de Camöes in *The Lusiads*, she is "a perfection of beauty [and] it must not be supposed that her intelligence was childish" (De Cervantes, 1605/1615, p. 618). But she let herself become enamoured of a guitar player, poet, and great dancer, very skilled at making birdcages. Decidedly, beards and cages haunt the novel, perhaps as surviving images of beards and cages from the bagnios of Algiers.

Using hackneyed oxymorons such as "in death I live, in ice I burn, in flames I shiver, hopeless I hope, I go and stay", the guitar-playing poet pierced the duena's heart, took advantage of her naivety, and worse still, turned her "senses [to] quicksilver" (De Cervantes, 1605/1615, p. 619). The consequences for the infanta in her charge were quick to emerge: "I perceived [...] a certain expansion of waist in Antonomasia."

Just as we say a Nero or a Don Quixote, we could call Antonomasias all maidens seduced by poets, whom the Distressed Duena wants to see "banished from all well-ordered States; at least the amatory ones, […] as Plato advised" (De Cervantes, 1605/1615, p. 619). It is obvious that the majordomo, author, actor, and director of this baroque opera, is a learned man.

Countess Doloride's recital ends with a catastrophic event that constitutes the high point of the drama. The lovers are united in matrimony, despite the disparity in their status. The princess's mother dies of a broken heart, although Sancho thinks there was no cause for this, since "of gentlemen knights, specially if they be errant, kings and emperors may be made" (De Cervantes, 1605/1615, p. 621).

But the real catastrophe is yet to come, more "bitter than colocynth". The lovers are changed into statues, she into an ape and he into "a horrible crocodile", by the giant Malambruno, who appeared, "mounted upon a wooden horse", over the queen's grave. Between the two statues, there stands a pillar—as stiff as the sword between Tristan and Isolda—with an inscription defying "the valiant Manchegan […] to do battle with me in single combat", in order to undo the enchantment.

And there is more. All at once, all the duenas "captained the veils with which they were covered, and disclosed countenances all bristling with beards, some red, some black, some white, and some grizzled" (De Cervantes, 1605/1615, p. 622). Don Quixote and Sancho have their work cut out for them. Now, they not only have to disenchant Dulcinea, but also the whole squadron of bearded duenas, who lament pitifully: "where […] can a duena with a beard [go] to? […] For, if even when she has a smooth skin, and a face tortured by a thousand kinds of washes and cosmetics, she can hardly get anybody to love her, what will she do when she shows a countenance turned into a thicket?"

Cervantes makes it a point to congratulate Cide Hamete, the Arab author, for overlooking no detail in his effort to "[make] plain the smallest points the most inquisitive can desire to know" (De Cervantes, 1605/1615, p. 623). This speaks volumes about the time he spent in his father's shop, where he learned the minute details related to the handling of beards.

Incidentally, the "bearded woman" was the nickname given to the heroine of *Celestina* (De Rojas, 1499), the first Spanish play, published at the opening of the sixteenth century, a play Cervantes knew by heart. The adjective was used to describe go-betweens who gained entry into households. By pretending to be cosmetics vendors, they smuggled love letters to young people. We note, in passing, the hair-removal technique still in use today, described by one of the bearded women: "we have [...] taken to using sticking plasters by way of an economical remedy, for by applying them to our faces and plucking them off with a jerk we are left as bare and smooth as the bottom of a stone mortar".

Don Quixote swears to do everything in his power to repair this physical and moral wrong: "I will pluck out my own [beard] in the land of the Moors, if I don't cure yours" (De Cervantes, 1605/1615, p. 623).

In the fourth act, a machine play will put an end to the duenas' enchantment.

Usque ad astra: to the stars

In logical fashion, the reader is taken from witchcraft to astrology, from the terrestrial microcosm to the heavenly macrocosm, which at the time fascinated Galileo, who built his telescope in 1609.

At the castle, a wooden horse was built in record time, reminiscent of Chevillard, the steed on which Pierres carried off the fair Magalona. This mount was to transport the two heroes to the far-away kingdom of Kandy.

No less imaginative than Leonardo da Vinci, Cervantes invents a flying horse that "neither eats nor sleeps nor wears out shoes". A much improved version of Pegasus, he "goes at an ambling pace through the air [...], so that he whom he has mounted upon him can carry a cup of water in his hand without spilling a drop" (De Cervantes, 1605/1615, p. 624). Who would be surprised at this today, when you can calmly sip a drink in mid-flight between Madrid and Colombo in Sri Lanka?

As for Sancho, he much prefers to stay on *terra firma*. His fear of bruising his backside if he rides "without pad or cushion" is probably a cover-up for fear of flying. He tries to refuse taking part in the mission by invoking the right to disobedience—an amendment made to France's Army regulations in 1975 (Barrois, 1993, p. 232), to be invoked when "orders are breaches to international law". According to Sancho, only the code of chivalry should govern voyages in outer space. "let each one shave himself as best he can; I'm not going to accompany my master on any such long journey".

And the tone goes up a notch, in a style imitating Figaro in *The Barber of Seville*: "In the king's name! What have squires got to do with the adventures of their masters? Are they to have the fame of such as they go through, and we the labor?"

Historians of the Annales School will appreciate the accent placed on the history of the people, rather than on the deeds of heroes.

> Body o' me! If the historians would only say, "Such and such a knight finished such and such an adventure, but with the help of so and so, his squire [...]"; but they write curtly, "Don Paralipomenon [...] accomplished the adventure of the six monsters", without mentioning such a person as his squire, who was there all the time, just as if there was no such being.
>
> (De Cervantes, 1605/1615, p. 625)

The irony is in the redundancy. Etymologically, Paralipomenon means "left out". In any case, "Help! Mayday!"—Sancho refuses to have anything to do with these bushy women, "from the highest to the lowest, and from the most prudish to the most affected" (De Cervantes, 1605/1615, p. 626). All these hairy things, "whiskered like infantrymen, scare the daylights out of [him]", as a bawdy French song says.

Horrible to behold! These possessors of the "Origin of the world", painted by Courbet and by Magritte with pubic beards, are ready to cut off what they do not possess. Ouch! Yet Sancho's terrible fear of castration is nothing compared to the trial awaiting him. At nightfall, "suddenly there came into the garden four wild men clad in green ivy bearing on their shoulders a great wooden horse" (De Cervantes, 1605/1615, p. 618), the famous steed Clavelino.

In the Middle Ages, wild men symbolised madness. Their domain was the space of the marvel, which, in this instance, will extend to intergalactic space, thanks to the surrealistic wooden horse. A forerunner of Swift's and Tristram Shandy's hobby horse, Clavelino also foreshadows the knights of the sky, with his wooden peg as a joy stick. He predates Cyrano's *A Voyage to the Moon* and Jules Verne's *From the Earth to the Moon*, as well as the inventions of Méliès, Hergé, creator of Tintin's *Objectif Lune*, and Saint Exupéry's *Little Prince* descended from his distant planet to befriend the stranded pilot.

This aircraft is as multifunctional as a Rafale fighter. To combat terrestrial or extraterrestrial monsters, it can fly at high or low altitude, and can hedgehop if the mission is to deforest all these mounds of Venus. It even flies higher, like a spaceship, where the extreme cold of upper spheres is followed by the fiery trajectory of descent upon re-entry into the atmosphere. In fact, Sancho worries about the duration of the return trip and about jet lag, as if he were being asked to embark on a trip to Mars: "[what] if [...] we'll be half a dozen years getting back" (De Cervantes, 1605/1615, p. 629).

In the end, he mounts on the croup of the steed, prompted not so much by the duke's supercilious deal that this voyage is to be "payment" for the promised government of an island (De Cervantes, 1605/1615, p. 629), but by rebellion against his master, who has the gall to ask him to give himself five hundred lashes "on account" before they leave, to disenchant Dulcinea. "By God, but your worship must be out of your senses! This is like the common saying, 'You see me with child and you want me a virgin'" (De Cervantes, 1605/1615, p. 630). But between two bad options, he chooses the lesser one: "Let us be off to shave these Duenas."

Unreason has triumphed over reason.

Flight simulator

The journey resembles a makebelieve voyage of initiation. Obliged to blindfold themselves to go through ordeals by fire and extreme cold, as in Mozart's *Magic Flute*, the two heroes are, in fact, the target of voyeurs who are laughing at them. What is the difference between an ancient mystery cult and this imposture, between symbolic efficiency and sterile deception, between the reader's salutary laugh and the manipulator's sniggering? No matter, for the masters of the collective fun-poking session become the dupes of their own deception when Don Quixote transforms the masquerade into a true scientific experiment: "Cover thine eyes, Sancho, and mount [...]; though all should turn out the contrary of what I hope, no malice will be able to dim the glory of having undertaken this exploit" (De Cervantes, 1605/1615, p. 632).

At first, the scenery resembles the scenes depicted in Flemish tapestries. "As [Don Quixote] had no stirrups and his legs hung down, he looked like nothing so much as a figure in some Roman triumph" (De Cervantes, 1605/1615, p. 630). Sancho has settled himself on the croup, sitting sideways, as in that way "he would not feel the hardness so much", according to the director of the play. In terms of special effects, the production team spared no effort, "the whole adventure was so well planned by the duke, the duchess, and their majordomo, that nothing was omitted to make it perfectly successful" (De Cervantes, 1605/1615, p. 632). Puffing with a great pair of bellows to produce strong wind, sound effects to imitate thunder and hail, fireworks and lightning for crossing thunder clouds, tow on the end of a reed set on fire to heat their faces … All the aerological phenomena are called into play.

Cervantes even invents the flight simulator. Instead of experiencing the event like a passive victim, his son achieves his dream of becoming a fighter pilot, elaborating a flight plan based on stories of flying fools, like the licentiate Torralba, arrested by the Inquisition in 1528 for having dreamt such dreams.

"The duke, the duchess, and all in the garden were listening to the conversation of the two heroes, and were beyond measure amused by it" (De Cervantes, 1605/1615, p. 632). Their technicians have filled the horse with "squibs and crackers", to which they now set fire with some tow applied to Clavileno's tail, so that the steed would take off like a spaceship on the launching pad at Cape Canaveral.

And the forerunner of Henri Farman, of Clément Ader, of Earth satellites and other Soyuz or Apollo spacecrafts, is sent off by the powerful breath of an out-of-control intelligence. Don Quixote has no doubt often observed the flight of birds; whirling buzzards carried by rising thermal currents, falcons able to gain very high altitudes and to sweep down "on the heron at three hundred kilometers an hour, so as to seize it however high it may soar", as well as the infallible flight instruments of migratory birds. He explains to his navigator the sensation of immobility in space, "one would fancy we never stirred from one place, [but] beyond a doubt, Sancho, we must have already reached the second region of the air" (De Cervantes, 1605/1615, p. 636).

Their landing, no less brutal than that of the Wright brothers in 1903 on the dunes of Cape Hatteras—after covering less than a hundred metres in their biplane—drives the hoax into the background, to focus on the passionate desire for space discoveries which, in Cervantes' time, produced Copernicus, Tycho Brahé, Kepler, and Galileo. Clavelino lands among people stretched on the ground, showing "wonder and amazement" as if they were coming out of a heavy sleep, reminiscent of the trance in the cave of Montesinos. An inscription on a parchment informs the heroes that the duenas, now disenchanted, have returned home.

But the joke falls flat during the debriefing stage of the mission, which acquires astronomical proportions, becoming as foolproof as the conquest of space.

Objectively speaking, when Sancho "drew aside the handkerchief covering [his] eyes ever so little, close to [his] nose", he should not have seen the earth "no bigger than a grain of mustard seed, and that the men walking on it were little bigger than hazel nuts" (De Cervantes, 1605/1615, p. 634). The duchess criticises his sense of proportion, unable—contrary to him—to imagine the splendour that would much later be described by astronaut Greg Chamitoff in electronic messages sent from the space station where he spent six months in 2008, and from which he took two spacewalks in 2011, during the last flight of the space shuttle *Endeavour*.

Sancho has journeyed in an astronaut's dream, among the goats of the Pleiades constellation—called "the seven she-goats" in Spanish. And he amused himself with them, for he had been a goat-herd as a child. "They did not care to ask him anything more about his journey, for they saw he was in the vein to go rambling all over the heavens giving an account of everything that went on there, without having ever stirred from the garden" (De Cervantes, 1605/1615, p. 635). Once again, Cervantes shows us how dreams and visions set the imagination in motion, both in science and in therapy. Don Quixote does not lose his wits either, and tells his squire in an aside: "Sancho, as you would have us believe what you saw in heaven, I require you to believe me as to what I saw in the cave of Montesinos; I say no more."

A word to the wise! This time, the message to be given to the forger consists in proving to him that journeys, even when they are made without moving from an office, a laboratory, or a prairie, are much more believable than his inept imitation.

In the second novel, the perspective of the knight has widened the field of research, expanding it from the inscription of war traumas all the way to perversion as a form of government.

Admonition

Seeing the Earth from Sirius—which was to be Voltaire's perspective in *Micromegas*—has transformed Sancho into a philosopher. He revises his ambitions: "what is there grand in being ruler of a grain of mustard seed?" A small bit of sky would be preferable, "if your lordship would be so good as to give [it to] me" (De Cervantes, 1605/1615, p. 636).

This might have been the beginning of star wars, had the duke not set everything in order by giving back to Caesar what is Caesar's, to

Sancho his pseudo-island, and the sky to God. So, Sancho accepts his terrestrial fate, curious "to try what it tastes like to be a governor" (De Cervantes, 1605/1615, p. 636). The duke assures him that once he has tasted governing, "you'll eat your fingers off after the government, so sweet a thing it is to command and be obeyed". The important thing is to be properly dressed for the position, "partly as a lawyer, partly as a captain, for, in the island I am giving you, arms are needed as much as letters, and letters as much as arms" (De Cervantes, 1605/1615, p. 637). The famous motto "The cowl does not make the monk", used by the duke as a slogan, is turned on its head by Sancho: "however I'm dressed I'll be Sancho Panza".

Now, Cervantes asks Don Quixote to teach a veritable lesson on governance. The knight takes his squire by the hand and brings him into his room; after closing the door and almost forcing Sancho to sit beside him, he develops the topic point by point, on the model of a medieval "Mirror for Princes".

First, a warning against the intoxicating effect of power: "attribute not the favor thou hast received to thine own merits". Woe to the one who believes himself to be all-powerful. Who has made you governor? You better know it, for tyrants, as we know, recruit among plotters and the very poor. The admonition is intended to keep Sancho's vanity in check: "First of all, my son, thou must fear God [...]. Secondly, thou must [...] know thyself"—*gnôthi seauton*—the Delphic maxim that, according to Socrates [Plato], recommends the most difficult thing [...] that the mind can imagine". Sancho must also keep in mind that "officers and great trusts are nothing else but a mighty gulf of troubles" (De Cervantes, 1605/1615, p. 638).

He must respect his ancestors, must not repudiate his humble origins, nor puff himself up like Aesop's frog: "Glory in the humble birth [...]; for when it is seen that thou art not ashamed no one will set himself to put thee to the blush [...]. If perchance anyone of thy kinfolk should come to see thee [...], thou art not to repel or slight him" (De Cervantes, 1605/1615, p. 638).

When Sancho is admonished not to forget that he once "kept pigs", he insists on pointing out that later he was promoted to keeping geese. Then, with no further ado, the knight issues an injunction regarding all first ladies: "[Carry] thy wife with thee ([for] it is not well for those that administer governments to be long without their wives), [...] strive to smooth down her natural roughness; for all that may be gained by a wise governor may be lost and wasted by a boorish stupid wife". Should he have to remarry, "if perchance thou art left a widower [...], choose not [a wife] to serve thee for a hook, or for a fishing rod". As for friends, "never go by arbitrary law, which is so much favored by ignorant men who plume themselves on cleverness" (De Cervantes, 1605/1615, p. 639).

After discussing God, lineage, marriage, and allies, the rhythm of Don Quixote's monologue brings to mind the balancing of the scales of justice. No demagogy: "Strive to lay bare the truth, as well amid the promises and presents of the rich man, as amid the sobs and entreaties of the poor." No corruption either: "press not the utmost rigor of the law against the guilty; [but] do not be swayed by the weight of a gift". Nor any resentment: "If it should happen thee to give judgment in the cause of one who is thine enemy, turn thy thoughts away from thy injury and fix them on the justice of the case." And beware of seduction: "If any handsome woman come to seek justice of thee, turn away thine eyes from her tears and thine ears from her lamentations, [...] if thou wouldst not have thine reason swept away by her weeping, and thy rectitude by her sighs." But, above all, no cruelty: "Abuse not by word him whom thou hast to punish in deed" (De Cervantes, 1605/1615, p. 639).

Here, Cervantes speaks from direct experience, recalling the abuses of power he has known both as a slave in Algiers and as a tax collector in Spain, when he found himself imprisoned in Seville, after the bank where he had deposited the money due to the Royal Treasury went bankrupt and the banker falsely accused him of dishonesty.

> If thou followest these precepts and rules, Sancho, thy days will be long, thy fame eternal, thy reward abundant, thy felicity unuttered; thou wilt marry thy children as thou wouldst; they and thy grandchildren will bear titles; [...] and, when life draws to a close, [...] the light and loving hands of thy great-grandchildren will close thine eyes.
>
> (De Cervantes, 1605/1615, p. 639)

The morality lesson is followed by practical advice, also rooted in the Middle Ages, when one's gestures and physical demeanour were as good as one's word.

The rationale of gestures

(J.-C. Schmidt, "The Rationale of Gestures in the West", in Bremmer and Roodenburg (Eds.), *A Cultural History of Gesture*. Cornell University Press, 1992).

The body reflects the soul. The future governor will have to cut his nails, because letting them grow like hawk claws is "a filthy and unnatural abuse" (De Cervantes, 1605/1615, p. 640). He is told not to wear loose clothes, for "disordered attire is a sign of an unstable mind". The liveries of his servants should be "respectable and serviceable, rather than showy and gay", and he should give the poor as many clothes as he gives his servants. He is advised not to eat garlic and onions, and to "walk slowly and speak deliberately, but not in such a way as to make it seem [he is] listening to [himself]". He is to dine sparingly and sup even more sparingly, and "be temperate in drinking, [for] wine in excess keeps neither secrets nor promises". He must not gorge himself, and must not "eruct".

Sancho does not know that "eruct" comes from the Latin and is used to avoid saying "to belch", "one of the filthiest words in [our] language" (De Cervantes, 1605/1615, p. 641). Don Quixote then moves from the language of bodily functions to language enrichment, "for custom will bring [words] into use in the course of time, so that they will be readily understood; this is the way a language is enriched; custom and the public are all powerful there".

It has become obvious since then that the life of language is constantly attacked by the "newspeak" of perverse systems (Orwell, 1950). In contrast, language enrichment through recourse to Latin and Arabic roots will be illustrated by the knight at the end of the novel. Sancho's contribution will consist in supplying a string of proverbs his master advises him not to "drag [...] in so often by the head and shoulders that they savor more of nonsense". But to Sancho, they are his literature, "His treasure of signifiers", as Lacan would say, his interpretation tool: "I have more proverbs in me than a book, and when I speak they come so thick together in my mouth [...] that my tongue lets fly the first that come, though they may not be pat to the purpose."

While Don Quixote is determined to tone down this passion for arts and crafts, Victor Hugo, an avid reader of the novel, drew inspiration from it:

> For words, let it be known, are living things,
> The dreamer's hand vibrates, trembles to write them;

> [...]
> Somber folk—so words come and go within us;
> They are the soul's mysterious passersby.
>
> (Hugo, 1859, pp. 177, 179)

After this flight of poetry, the advice becomes more practical again. First, the manner of sitting on a horse, so as to have the mien of a gentleman, instead of sitting so loosely "that one would suppose thou wert on Dapple" (De Cervantes, 1605/1615, p. 641). Then, no sleeping in, "for he who does not rise early does not get the benefit of the day". Finally, a last bit of Cervantian wisdom is passed down to Sancho: "The last counsel I will give thee now, though it does not tend to bodily improvement, [...] is this—never engage in a dispute about families, at least in the way of comparing them one with another."

There can be no doubt that the reader is admonished to remember the quixotic mantra that "all comparison is offensive".

The art of the proverb

Sancho, who has been able to remember only the first two admonitions—not letting his nails grow and remarrying if he becomes widowed—asks that all this advice be put in writing, although he does not know how to read or write. In fact, in order to hide this, he will pretend his right hand is disabled (De Cervantes, 1605/1615, p. 642)—like the left hand of the famous one-armed man from Lepanto—and will lose the list his master wrote out for him almost as soon as he gets it.

The theme of the lost letter is reiterated, awakening echoes of another lost manuscript, encountered at the start of the first novel (De Cervantes, 1605/1615, p. 50). His master's advice was going to re-emerge in the governor's mind, as faithfully conserved as his cherished proverbs.

The art of speaking in proverbs, as witnessed by Jean Paulhan (1993) in Madagascar, consists in making use of them appropriately in a discussion, to dispel confusion, or to make a clear decision. New at this exercise that is "inflicting the pangs of torture on [him]", Don Quixote asks his squire: "How dost thou apply them, thou blockhead?"

The value of the wisdom of nations, like that of all language games, Wittgenstein would say, lies in the use that is made of it. This skill for proper application is Sancho's only valuable possession: "Why the devil should you be vexed if I make use of what is my own? And I have got nothing else, nor any other stock in trade except proverbs and more proverbs."

Magnanimously, Don Quixote asks him to quote two or three that come to his mind, "pat to the purpose and like pears in a basket". Four maxims come to Sancho's mind on the spot, to express his conception of the founding principle of politics: "While we're asleep we're all equal."

Consequently, he is no longer so keen to govern, "for I know no more about the government of islands than a buzzard", and is ready to forget the whole thing: "Senor, if your worship thinks I'm not fit for this government, I give it up on the spot; for the mere black of of the nail on my soul is dearer to me than my whole body" (De Cervantes, 1605/1615, p. 644).

The selflessness to which these words testify is the trait Bion attributed to the true leader in a leaderless group (1961). Hearing them, Don Quixote tells Sancho: "I consider thou deservest to be governor of a thousand islands. Thou hast good natural instincts, without which no knowledge is worth anything."

This statement echoes Gargantua's letter to his son Pantagruel, who is about to leave to study in Paris (Rabelais, c. 1532–1564): "Science without conscience is the soul's perdition." Sancho has passed the recruitment test, based on the slightly daft criterion of the foolishness linking him to his master, which, paradoxically, endows him with discernment. A word to the wise! The man lifted from the ranks has stepped beyond the Mirror of Vanities, and proclaims his credo: "I was born naked and I will die naked!"

After the encounter with the Theatre of Death a few chapters earlier, a true *ars moriendi* is initiated. Determined that his hero, Don Quixote, must die—so that no forger may write a sequel to his adventures—Cervantes forces us to start thinking about the immortal hero's death, while he prepares for his own and prepares us for ours. His frequent brushes with death lead him to the conclusion that a man's last steps in life are a source of vitality for his grandchildren.

In contrast, the ducal couple wants to reap the benefits of its fools' vitality, lest it be stricken with sloth. Called *acedia* in the Middle Ages, and considered a sin (Jéquier, 2001, p. 53), this apathy is associated with self-love, and evokes our postmodern depression, obsessed with itself.

In order to feed on the vital energy of his two jesters, the duke attacks their *philia* by separating them surgically. The aim of this experimental protocol is to destroy Sancho's soul, in a village the duke possesses, called, for the sake of the joke, the island of Barataria. The name brings to mind Barathrum, the mythological abyss of Hell. In French, *baratin* means "blah blah blah".

While Sancho is on his way to the pseudo-government of his fake island, Cervantes, through the mouth of Cide Hamete, apologises to the reader for having bored him with two dull chapters on principles of moral conduct. His only excuse is that he resisted his own penchant for digression—much criticised in the first novel—and kept his imagination in check, "[restricting] himself to the narrow limits of the narrative".

This rigorous constraint produced, in the book we are reading, an art of fugue and counterpoint, where the adventures of the two heroes will become intertwined thanks to the distance between them. Still, the plural body that ensures their survival will make use of this splitting to escape from the deadly schemes that are being plotted against them.

Dismembering the plural body

In the meantime, they are both made anxious by Sancho's departure. Without knowing it, they have sensed the escalation of violence that thrills the audience.

Sancho is sent off to govern his island, escorted by the duke's major-domo, "a man of great discretion and humour". But he confides to his master that he recognised at once the face of the Distressed Countess when he saw him. Don Quixote agrees, but he warns his squire that "this is not the time for going into questions of the sort, which would be involving ourselves in an inextricable labyrinth" (De Cervantes, 1605/1615, p. 646). Wise advice! The reader is also warned not to waste his energy if he ever finds himself in a similar situation. Still, Sancho remains "on the lookout" and promises to tell his master what he discovers. Even if their messages are intercepted by the ducal intelligence services, what is essential will never be uncovered, for it pertains to another kind of discourse that has nothing to hide, as Erasmus claims in his *Praise of Folly*.

Here, Cervantes presents his analysis of the invisible causes of the country's decadence. Thanks to his ties to the business world, he understands the economic situation analysed forty years ago by historian Pierre Vilar (1971). A hostile attitude to emerging capitalism leads to the expulsion of Jewish financiers and Muslim merchants. Yet the pillage perpetrated in the New World is supplying Europe with precious metals that generate profits, above all, for German and Genoise bankers. At the same time, Spain accumulates debt, rejecting investment and savings.

In all classes of Spanish society, the ratio of those who work compared to those who do not is one in thirty. There is terrible poverty, the plague is devastating the population, inflation is ruining the merchants and craftsmen who stayed in the country, and who come to be despised by the idle classes at both ends of the social spectrum. At the top, the very rich like the ducal couple, and at the bottom those who belong to the criminal underworld of picaresque novels, sing the praises of a life of leisure, each in his own way. In fact, Spain became bankrupt four times in the Golden Age, and had to issue copper coins at the turn of the seventeenth century.

"The century is truly devastating", Cervantes proclaims, because it leads the country into a long sleep. *Otium versus negotium*! Sloth triumphs over work and commerce. Does this mean that some must work so that the rest can be idle? Must there be children who are slaves in far-off lands so that our children can be consumers of cheap goods? To raise this question, the duke's emissaries send real rogues to Sancho's judgement seat. Each time, he transforms the joke played on him into a case illustrating ethical and political principles.

The success of the Second Part of *Don Quixote* is due in part to the fact that it reveals the moral disintegration under the ducal regime of hyperactivity. Moreover, it proposes possible answers instead of announcing the end of the world. Cervantes criticises the fascination of the elite with the shady world of picaros, no doubt familiar to him. Still, the horizons he wants to open for the reader are not those of the underworld where the rich seek their thrills, but rather the open spaces of freedom.

A word to the wise! Cervantes transforms the decay of the social link into fertile ground where poetry can bloom, like the literary epitaphs offered, in his first novel, to his fallen war buddies without graves (De Cervantes, 1605/1615, p. 58). Now, his task is to teach us to leave the regions of death, instead of "lapping them up and licking our fingers", as Swift writes in his "Digression on madness" (1704). From the two separate places where Don Quixote and Sancho now find themselves, literally disfigured and stomped upon, their voices will speak in unison, bequeathing to the reader a revitilising energy passed down for centuries.

This refusal of voluntary submission is held up as an example in a Lope de Vega play brought by a patient to his analyst in a moment of madness.

CHAPTER FOUR

Fuenteovejuna

Resisting together

Unexpectedly, a man comes to his session with a little book for the analyst. By this time, the analysis has reached a point of palpable tension for both of them. On the cover of the book, under the name of Lope de Vega (1618), the analyst reads *Fuenteovejuna*, a play written about the time of Cervantes' death and published a few years later.

The prefatory notice explains that *Fuenteovejuna* is a play based on actual historic events that took place in Spain in 1476, in a village called Fuenteovejuna. An officer, Fernan Gomez de Guzman, mistreated the villagers cruelly, until the day they banded together and killed him. King Ferdinand II of Aragon sent a magistrate to investigate the murder. When he arrived in the village, the magistrate questioned the villagers one after the other, asking: "Who killed Don Fernan?" Despite threats and torture, all the villagers responded only by saying: "Fuenteovejuna did it."

Background: Spain is entering a turbulent period in its history. A few years earlier, Isabella of Castile and Ferdinand of Aragon married, in order to unite their two kingdoms. But Alphonse V of Portugal crossed into Spain in order to secure the throne for Juana, daughter of the deceased king Enrique. Alphonse V suffered a decisive defeat in the battle of Toro in 1474, two years before the incident in Fuenteovejuna.

The war was ferocious and continued to be waged among different factions. What was at stake was the very legitimacy of power. Some one hundred and fifty years later, Lope de Vega, at the height of his success, wrote a story of treason, sexual abuse, abuse of power, cruelty, and resistance, which ended with the pardon granted by the Catholic monarchies henceforth united in equal legitimacy, as the well-known motto indicates: *Tanto monta, monta tanto, Isabel como Fernando* (It makes no difference, it's all the same, Isabella or Fernando).

Isabella and Ferdinand ascended to the throne, each of them in turn, with rights recognised as equal. They granted their pardon to the village of Fuenteovejuna, acknowledging the value of its resistance when it refused to be divided, to break its bond of solidarity in the face of the judicial investigation attempting to identify the murderer. The village carried out its own justice against a brutal and perverse officer.

This lesson in resistance, recognised and celebrated by the writer, was the one the patient chose to bring to the analyst at a crucial and difficult point in their relationship.

The analyst took the little book, unaware of the huge effort the patient would still have to make to force him to enter into the context and content of his story, intertwined with History, to lead their sessions and their interaction to the point where inscription, and even writing, become possible.

The walls have ears

Especially when there is no one to hear, when fear reigns supreme. The analyst had first seen this man, a little older than himself, about thirty years ago. From the start, given the distraught state in which the first session had left him, the analyst decided to see him now only once a week, on Wednesday afternoons. The sessions had to be at least two hours long, and the analyst left them in such a state that his two children, who had no school on Wednesday afternoons, needed about two hours to bring their father back to himself and to the more poetic side of life. It took all this time for him to recover his ability to play with them, and recover the joy that went with it.

Indeed, this patient had drawn him mercilessly into the heart of his delusion, which apparently left him no rest. He was constantly observed by agents of the secret police, who followed him, listened in on his phone calls, and even tried to guess his thoughts. First, the analyst tried to assure him that their sessions were safe and confidential. When he told him that there were no microphones hidden in the walls or between the books, this tortured man only smiled tensely, giving him a knowing look. He pointed to the analyst's watch, saying that it must be hiding a microphone and an antenna, which transmitted their conversations to all the police cars. The analyst took off his watch and lent it to him, aware that fire trucks and ambulances drove by constantly, since their sirens made it hard to ignore them. His office was near three hospitals and a fire station.

The tension kept mounting. One day, at his wits' end, the analyst ended up telling the patient that it was hard enough to understand his complex deductions, without imagining that someone else would bother to listen to them repeatedly on recordings, even out of curiosity. This comment made the patient smile again, perhaps less nervously. Afterwards, it seemed as if they had carved out together a space of temporary safety, wrested from the continuity of the delusion, but which did not extend beyond the analyst's office, to provide any further protection in the patient's everyday life.

A few months before their first meeting, he had spent quite a long time in a psychiatric hospital; using a screwdriver and a hammer, he had knocked out several of his teeth. It was the only way he had found to get rid of the microphones that had mysteriously been implanted in his mouth, in his body.

Collaboration, political purge: an eight-year-old witness

In their fragile weekly refuge, the patient was able to give some indication of what his childhood had been like. The analyst listened carefully, but was lifted out of his chair by the constant use of the present tense. He was in the midst of it all. Right there in his office, the Second World War was unfolding. And all the themes of the patient's delusions suddenly fell into place.

He was born a few years before the war, in a bourgeois family running a luxury shop in a chic area of Paris. He remembered clearly the look of the German officers who had become the rich clients of the store under the Occupation. He also remembered the special treatment at the butcher's shop: the women lined up with their food ration tickets, while his mother quickly came out of the shop with a package of meat, and went off with him under the furious stares of the other women.

But most importantly, he was there when the police knocked on their door one day, early in the morning, a few weeks after the end of the war. A joyful and profitable period of collaboration for some was followed by a dark period of purge, often carried out by the same protagonists, who had lost no time before changing sides.

That morning, while he is still in bed, he hears the noise and confusion when the plain-clothes men burst in. Then a long silence. He understands that his father left with the police captain. They come back an hour later. His father shouts to his wife: "Give them everything!" He no doubt meant the gold, accumulated and hidden during the profitable period of trade with the Germans.

The child had stayed in his bed. At this point, he takes the time to summarise the situation to a few short formulas which, the patient tells the analyst, are still as hard-hitting now as they were then. His father's absence for an hour after the knocking on the door was registered as: "A hole in the ass in the police captain's office." His father was fucked by the police in exchange for his freedom. His mother was a whore, she sold her favours to the butcher for a piece of meat. Everything comes together to confirm what he believes; his conviction is unshakable.

The analyst can easily imagine the insults and jeering that his parents had to face in the following weeks: "She was the Germans' whore"; "It serves him right, they fucked him in the ass!" Resounding with shame and dishonour, the words are stripped of the colourful veneer conferred by their use in street slang: they become projectiles that wound or kill every time. There is no more room for metaphors: the world is filled with sound and fury, with compact signs. Time itself has become compact. No reconstitution is helpful for interpreting. Any attempt at explanation turns into an embarrassing error.

This was the world in which the child grew up, went to school, living henceforth in a family with limited means. He became an adult, married and divorced, but in fact always remained frozen in that moment which had pushed him into the margins of time. Frozen in fear, shame, and the knowing silence attached to them. In any event, his questions, his attitudes, and his suspicions became increasingly unbearable for his family, which wanted only to forget and regain its status, like many others at the time.

His mother was striving to see her daughters recover their splendour of bygone days. She succeeded, through relations and intrigues, to find them husbands belonging to families of bankers who had collaborated almost openly with the enemy. As for him, he remained alone. One day, beside herself, she remarked scornfully: "You have always been the worst of my daughters!" Following the logic of the events which "cleared" his father, which he saw as prostitution, he was convinced that the sharing and transmission of power takes place between men through actual homosexual relations from which, once again, he felt excluded.

Caligraphy in the psychiatric hospital

A few months after his first visit to the analyst, a major crisis arose. He intended to spend a few days, while on vacation, in a family home in the south of France, in the middle of a sprawling domain which had belonged to his great-grandfather. The latter had amassed a fortune in South America. The patient had known him well and had fond memories of him, since he had been the only person in the world who invented games they could play together; he built small toys for him using bits of wood, nails, and string. "They never came out right", he added almost joyfully.

One morning, it was clear that his family could no longer bear his comments and his veiled but violent threats. They called the psychiatric emergency service in the nearest town, without telling him. Two nurses in civilian clothes entered the house and told him firmly to come with them; they left in the emergency vehicle, sirens blaring. In the rear-view mirror, he could see a car following them closely, until they were in a large courtyard: no doubt his father's car.

So he found himself in the hospital again, for a few days. But he had had time to take his great-grandfather's diary. It was a small notebook, handwritten, a "household accounts" book, as they used to be called, written in uncial script. During his hospital stay, he read over and over his ancestor's adventures in America: his return, his parrot, his Indian wife, the purchase of the domain, his remarriage, the gossip, and so on.

It took several more weeks for the analyst to be told of all this, and for him to try to understand the sequence of events. The message was constantly confused by interferences coming from a universal plot, which now extended to the therapist and his own associations, although the space of their meetings seemed to resist and survive. However, outside violence raged. His ferocious desire to break the sexual exclusion preventing him from having access to the powers shared by men pushed him to seek out male prostitutes in the streets, and he had been attacked several times after these paid encounters.

The social link established through prostitution reached its peak when it started to invade his work as a teacher. At one point, he became convinced that when a girl was late for school, it meant that she had been prostituted with the complicity of the school administration in the underground parking lot of the school. The teenage girl's troubled expression was a clear sign of sexual abuse, and the note signed by the school monitor was concrete proof of a universal criminal plot.

The analyst was losing hope of ever being able to reach the compact core of the patient's delusion. At the same time, he was aware that he was himself resisting with all his might, to protect the fragile space of their sessions—no doubt, also in order to protect himself as best he could. And it was then that the analyst's resistance gave way, broken by events he could have neither foreseen nor controlled.

A letter, a date

What was it that the patient could have spotted, in his frenzy, in the stability of the weekly setting and the relative safety it provided, due to microscopic changes that only the most amazing acuity could discern? In any case, one day he came to the session without the usual painful armour of his delusion, armed only with Lope de Vega's play as a gift for the analyst. Of course, in his quest for a power to which he felt he had always been refused access, he emphasised this equal alliance between a man and a woman, seen as constituting the new legitimacy of Catholic monarchs. But the analyst was more interested in the story of the resistance of this little village to the aggressor, and its courage in not denouncing the murderer or murderers of the tyrant, despite threats and torture, but simply repeating in unison the name of their village. This man, who spoke Spanish perfectly, insisted on the tone of voice of the choir of villagers, the *voz ronca*, a husky voice relying on the internal force of this resistance shown by all and by each one.

One week later, still in this unusual paranthesis, he informed the analyst that he had spent hours and whole days at the National Library, copying lines from ancient manuscripts. He wanted to feel in his hand the shape of the cursive script in his great-grandfather's diary. He showed the analyst a sheet of paper on which he had written his own name in this script: one could see certain features of it clearly, like the ∂ ending at the top in a descending curve, or the same letter **V** used to designate both the ***U*** and the *V*. It was uncial script.

That night, the analyst had a strange dream. He was a child, playing in a square of the city where he was born during the war: the Square of Peace. In the dream, he saw himself on one side of the square, before a white wall on which the names of fallen soldiers were carved in black. In the middle of the wall, a gigantic woman with a solemn look, in black bronze, wearing a headdress resembling the one seen on the coins of that era, stood with her arms extended in a cross-like posture. Under her right arm appeared the names of the men fallen in the First World War; under her left arm, the names of the men killed in the Second World War.

Above her head, a commemorative inscription spoke of mourning and gratitude: MACON TO HER CHILDREN FALLEN FOR FRANCE. The inscription was written in the Latin uncial script widely used on monuments, and resembled the patient's great-grandfather's handwriting.

In the dream, the child in the square was reading, calling out each letter separately, impressed by the long list of the fallen, FALLEN FOR FRANCE. He was reading POVRE (poor) instead of "POVR" (for), not aware of the spelling at that age. There could be no mistake, "poor France", as people said then, to have lost so many of her children in these two wars, the last one still so recent. After all, his own father's name could have appeared among the names under the huge left arm of the statue.

When he awakened, this reading by the child provided a precise historical point of reference, constituting the message the dream tried to deliver. This hesitant way of reading meant that the analyst could not have been more than three or four years old, when he was learning the alphabet and the rudiments of reading at the nearby nursery school.

As for the end of the Second World War, the child did not have any particular traumatic memories; but he remembered quite clearly July 14th 1945, when he was a little more than two years old. He knew, because he had been told, that the city had suddenly been invaded by the Germans, and that the militia reigned supreme in the city. Between 1942 and 1945 (the analyst was born in 1943), his father had lived the clandestine life of an escaped prisoner of war, and what's more, married to the daughter of a Jewess ostensibly named Levy, who had always refused to wear the yellow star and flee the city in the 1940 exodus. Thus, his father had been exposed to the risk of being denounced, of being sent off to some work camp, or worse. It was much later, no doubt prompted by the transference with this patient, that the analyst was able to reconstitute a remarkable event that had taken place in his native town under the Occupation: doctor Leon Israel, a close friend of his grandmother's, was killed in his home by the militia, and had a burial attended by an immense crowd of people who came to pay tribute to him, in the face of the Gestapo. Indeed, the funeral procession had been a silent act of resistance, fists clenched in open defiance, in 1944. The analyst was one year old then, and had kept the often-mentioned event in the shadows of his prehistory.

After having dreamt these very precise details, he reflected on this reading, U/V, which opened onto the suffering of a whole nation, even though a large portion of it had quickly resigned itself to collaborationist neutrality, while the population was busy finding daily sustenance. Of course, this sombre political context could not have been clear to a child of three or four. Therefore, the analyst started to reconstruct the reality of those times based on books written by rigorous historians. Those sombre times, both politically and morally, constituted the period when his city, his family, and himself were living through the early period of his life.

The analyst recounted this dream to the patient, since the dream had been triggered by the reading of uncial script after the patient had shown him his name written in this script, on a sheet of paper. The patient seemed a little surprised; still, the account of the dream seemed to provide him with some respite in the midst of the clamour of the terrifying messages that continued to assail him.

Writing, inscription

Indeed, the institution where he was teaching had become nothing more than a permanent sound box for his delusions. The latest developments pierced his body and mind without encountering any obstacle. His pupils, surprised at first, were now making fun of him openly, watching for his sudden, unjustified silences in the middle of a lesson, interrupted at times by tears and sobbing. The analyst was on the point of looking for some means of protection that seemed urgently needed.

On that very day, the man started his session in a particularly dramatic way: in tears, he told the analyst what had happened recently to one of his students. The girl had been very late coming to class, she had even had to see the school nurse first, and she brought him a certificate to prove it. No doubt, she had been sexually assaulted in the underground parking, had to receive medical care after being raped, and now he was handing the analyst the stamped memo to prove the criminal treatment to which the girl had been subjected. Standing, in tears, he insisted: "Here, this is proof of what I have been saying for so long. It's written on this paper. Take it! And keep it!"

The analyst took the sheet of paper that was folded in four and placed it near the telephone. For the rest of the session, they talked about countless other things. The week passed without the analyst giving any further thought to the famous piece of paper. Suddenly, on the morning of the next session, he remembered the paper. He spent over an hour looking for it in every corner, under the books and documents on his desk. But the piece of paper had vanished. Fearing the reaction this treacherous act perpetrated by local enchanters might trigger on the part of the patient, he started to prepare an explanation: a gust of wind, the vacuum cleaner, a terrible mistake that led to throwing the paper in the wastebasket…

As for the patient, he arrived on time. Very calm. His face, usually contorted, had changed, and his relaxed features were almost unrecognisable. His first words, spoken without anxiety, were: "Do you think that I will ever return to the psychiatric hospital?" The analyst was so surprised by this change of vertex, as Bion would say, which showed that this man could look at madness from the outside, that he completely forgot about the loss of the piece of paper. But how to connect the disappearance of the delusion with the disappearance of the paper without being delusional?

The fact is that the delusion never returned. The analyst's erasure—which apparently went back to his early childhood—of the denunciations, the denials, the threats that were part of the reality of the early post-war era in which he had found himself at the most tender age, had been rekindled by a dream. This dream had clearly sprung from the transference which had concentrated all that was essential into the shape of a single letter and opened the way for the cut-out unconscious of the analyst's first years of life. Yes, he and his patient had shared the same circumstances, the same atmosphere. Like all children, they had

had to construct interpretations as best they could, in order to account for events so mysterious, secret, and violent. His mistake of losing the document attesting to the entire plot evoked that terrible time when half of France accused the other half of having collaborated with the enemy, and when some people, in charge of sorting through the denunciations, had chosen to throw them in the waste paper basket. Not to deny what almost everyone knew, but in order to show mercy for their poor, torn country.

This is how it had been possible to resolve this type of transference, through the loss of confidential documents disclosing the secret of collusion in plain sight, thereby opening a space of new potential. But these things will continue to exist no matter what you do, reasonable men will tell us. In this case, let the form of a single letter serve as our support. We can nevertheless call "inscription" the process that resulted in the disappearance of the delusion. The inscription in the text of history of crucial and painful moments no longer required that testimony continue to be brought again and again in the present. It became possible to forget—that is, to remember as well—the passages censure had erased, the names endlessly repeated, the facts that were denied, and even the confusion of genders.

The analyst had kept for himself the connections triggered by his childhood memory of confusing the U and the V, and had never mentioned the word "inscription" to his patient. But as we know, these determined investigators are the rigorous theoreticians of our erasures. After a few months, during which both enjoyed the serenity of interesting, cordial conversation, the patient decided to end their weekly meetings.

He arrived for his last session with a little package he opened in the analyst's office. He had wished to bring as a gift an object from his home. At first, he thought of a big toothed wheel, threatening-looking gears he had stored in his attic. But on second thought, what he took out of the wrapping paper was a "writing box" made of brass. Consisting of a long pen-case and an ink-well attached to a base, it was the kind of object that the messengers of the sultans of the Ottoman Empire wore around their waists while they rode on their horses through the provinces, sent from Istanbul with directives from the Sublime Porte. Thanks to this device, they were always ready to write and sign ordinances to be carried out immediately.

The analyst accepted the gift. Nothing could have been better suited for signing an "inscription". The writing box is still on a shelf in his office. He wrote these lines, no doubt connected to the writing instrument of the Turks. This man's participation in what became a text a quarter of a century later is undeniable. In the end, the analyst had to recognise in the endurance of these symptoms the resistance of History itself to bringing the truth to light.

Thirty years later …

… Another dream arrived to validate these lines. Once he put away his pen, his "writing box", the analyst felt happy to have resuscitated these old memories. And the night brought him a new tell-tale dream, more than twenty years later.

In the dream, he was in his native town, as an adult this time. In fact, for many years, he had gone there only rarely. But in the dream, he wanted to show his wife the neighbourhood where he grew up. It was a pleasant neighbourhood, between the Saône and the police headquarters, no doubt renovated after he had left town at eight and a half years of age.

He and his wife are walking together towards the analyst's grandmother's apartment, inside what was left of an eighteenth-century mansion house. Surprise! Where all the newer buildings surrounding the house used to be, the space had been completely cleared. One could still see the traces of the excavators and demolition equipment. All that was left, in all its splendour, was this odd house with its stone staircase. Everything was gleaming brightly in the light of the sunset. In place of the tiny inner courtyards, there were now gardens as far as the eye could see Versailles! Through the window above the stone sink in the kitchen, one could even see mountains gleaming in the distance. Fortunately for us, there are dreams which set up mountains on the horizon of the flattest plains! It was too much, as children like to say, and the analyst was now showing his wife the enchanted land he had sometimes talked about, but always with some critical distance.

However, this palatial structure, this "folly", as it was called in the seventeenth and eighteenth centuries, was surrounded, in this dream landscape, by a double railing sculpted in white marble. At eye level, a frieze bore complicated motifs of seashells, flowers, and serpentine plants. In his dream, the analyst took a piece of the sculpture between his fingers: it broke into pieces. The whole thing was made of pasteboard.

Celestina: remember the madam!

We are back in the pasteboard ducal castle. The attack on the link has produced its effects. After Sancho's departure, Don Quixote is subject to a bout of despair, giving the impression that the scheme will succeed. We are reminded of acts of vandalism, which destroy the symbols of others, their gods, their idols. Soul murder covers up actual murder (Caviness, 2003, pp. 99–114). The two heroes are in danger of losing their vital energy.

A small detail points to the depletion suffered by the knight after the loss of his squire. Back in his room after they had taken leave of each other "with tears", Don Quixote again refuses the Duchess' offer that "four of my damsels, as beautiful as flowers, shall wait upon you" (De Cervantes, 1605/1615, p. 647). Obviously, the great lady identifies more and more with the madam, Celestina, who ushered in the picaresque literary aesthetic.

Cervantes knew by heart the discourse of the old "bearded woman", a pitiful, oppressed victim of the system she unscrupulously exploited. Her rhetoric in defence of the victimised beguiles Calisto—Melibea's faint-hearted, bashful suitor—and manipulates him for financial gain. The two lovers pay with their lives the old ogre's intrusion into their love affair.

Celestina starts by literally gaining entry into Melibea's home to fill the place left free by the mistress of the house. Although she is aware of the danger, the young girl's mother goes out to take care of the poor, just at the moment when the madam enters. The intrusion of the prostitutive social link drains the lovers' dreams of their substance, and eventually leads to their deaths: Calisto's first, then that of his young valets after Celestina's murder, and finally that of Melibea, who throws herself from a tower at her father's feet. The play closes with the latter's lamentations over his daughter's corpse.

Many critics of the last century had a very favourable view of the portrayal of this rebellious character taking power away from the patriarchal authorities of the city. Yet the author, Fernando de Rojas, a converted Jew, introduced the play by presenting it "as warning of the deceptions and tricks of procuresses", and "a caution to crazed lovers [...] overcome by their immoderate appetites" (De Rojas, 1499). Why not believe him instead of always looking for a subtext, as is so often done with *Don Quixote*? (Arrabal, 1996). Presuming that the writing is coded is a way to present the author as superior to the reader who simply loves a masterpiece.

A century after Rojas, Cervantes invents a Celestinian duchess to whom the hero successfully resists thanks to his candour. Don Quixote refuses again to be stripped naked by the madam's girls. He prefers to "sleep in

[his] own clothes, sooner than allow anyone to undress [him]", and he declares that he wants to wait upon himself. No one other than Sancho shall touch him. Playing the perfect hostess, the duchess concedes and offers to provide him with "all the utensils requisite" to spend the night alone in his room. Now he is at his own mercy, and anguish overtakes him when he finds himself alone after dinner and hears "a burst, not of sighs [...], but of some two dozen stitches in one of his stockings, that made it look like a window lattice" (De Cervantes, 1605/1615, p. 648).

The shameful grid of his forefathers' prisons is transformed into a lack of green silk for which he "would have given an ounce of silver, as if he tumbled down the social scale to the lowest picaresque rung". Here, Cide Hamete alludes to the precariousness which forces men of good birth to dine "miserably and in secret, and [make] a hypocrite of the toothpick [...], fancying they perceive a league off the patch on his shoe, the sweat stains on his hat, the shabbiness of his cloak, and the hunger in his stomach!" (De Cervantes, 1605/1615, p. 648).

But Cervantes believes the melancholia of the knight to be due less to his poverty than to the absence of his *therapon*. "A single being is missing, and everything is unpeopled!" (De Lamartine, 1993) says the poet. The burst stitches lay out the knight's distress all over his leg. When the plural body breaks up, when self-esteem comes undone as easily as the stitches in one's stockings, Celestinas hasten, with their scurrying gait, to turn this moment to their advantage.

Don Quixote's room on the first floor is perfect for the staging of a scene from the *corral de comedias*, a courtyard theatre specific to the Spanish Golden Age, which still exists in the Spanish town of Almagro. The two-tier stage allows for asides, "words under one's breath", mumbled by Celestina between her teeth—though she no longer had them. At the lower level, two fourteen-year-old maidens sent by the Duchess, Altisidora, and her pal Emerencia, are determined to give the knight a hell of a time. He, on his upper level, "to let them know he was there [...] gave a pretended sneeze, at which the damsels were not a little delighted". Thus, Don Quixote listened to their serenade, an amused ode to the male body under the coat of arms:

> O for to be the happy fair
> Thy mighty arms enfold,
> Or even sit beside thy bed
> And scratch thy dusty poll!
>
> (De Cervantes, 1605/1615, p. 651)

Although he is tickled by the prank, Don Quixote shut his window, "as much out of temper and out of sorts as if some great misfortune had befallen him" (De Cervantes, 1605/1615, p. 652). He has grasped their mockery and scolds them for persecuting Dulcinea, compared to whom these damsels are "ill-favored, foolish, light and low-born". Less than fifteen years old, by complying with their mistress's orders to excite the chaste knight, they are following the path charted by Celestina.

When the bearded woman leaves Areusa's house after instructing the girl to debauch Parmeno, she licks her gums, she says, to savour the aftertaste of the sexual encounter she forced her young recruit to have against her will (De Rojas, 1499). The boy's initiation takes place in the wings, but a rape has actually taken place on the stage earlier, when the old procuress, after taking pleasure at the sight of Areusa's naked body, intrudes into her womb to check if the cause of her pain is a pregnancy caused by a previous lover.

The two Celestinas, Rojas and Cervantes, feast on innocence by pushing young girls to debauchery. To avoid falling into this trap, Don Quixote invokes Dulcinea. But, clearly, his transferential apparatus is not at its best, since he has been separated from his squire. Now we wonder what misfortunes will befall Sancho, the duchess's favourite fool?

And He elevates the humble! Neither dissenter nor reactionary, Cervantes is not advocating the establishment of a new order. He is exploring the unrest of a society from which he himself tried to escape several times. First, by fleeing to Italy in his youth, and after returning from the bagnios, by attempting to sail to the West Indies. His requests for overseas positions, such as that of governor of Soconusco in Guatemala, *corregidor* in La Paz, or royal treasurer of the kingdom of New Grenada, were probably refused because they were reserved for "Old Christians" (Allendesalazar, 2004, p. 293).

Thus, Sancho would become governor in his place. He would be spared none of the humiliations to which Cervantes himself had been subjected. Despite the duke's plan to have him treated like the idiot described by the counterfeiter, the pseudo-governor would succeed in turning the mirror of madness against his aggressor.

Sotties

The mock trials enacted in Sotties are perfectly illustrated by the three cases presented to the new governor immediately upon his arrival.

Today, the plaintiffs would arouse sympathy among the defenders of various causes. But Sancho dismantles their schemes, demonstrating that they are the swindlers. The offended woman is revealed to be greedy, the abused old man is a crook, and the robbed buyer is as much a rogue as the seller.

In these three cases, the squire's wise judgement relies on the seismograph of his impressions, giving gestures the value of words. The power of powerlessness! Although Sancho does not know how to read, he is experienced in unmasking disguises, and he perceives their unconscious gestures on the stage of the trial (Felman, 2002).

The tailor and his client are both dismissed, for having tried to trick each other. The cane of the poor old man, handed to the lender while the first man swears that he gave back the money, turns out to be the hiding place for the stolen money. The outraged woman demonstrates publicly that she is very capable of protecting her most valuable possession. When, on Sancho's orders, her patsy tries to get back the money awarded by the judge, she defends the purse, held against her belly, with such strength that the man cannot take it from her.

Indeed, the governor triumphs over the treacherous intentions of those who attempt to ridicule him.

"Rough music" at the castle

In the meantime, Don Quixote is severely wounded on the face by a great sack full of cats, "which [...] had bells [...] tied to their tails", and "a cord with more than a hundred bells attached to it" (De Cervantes, 1605/1615, p. 664).

Traditionally, "rough music" (Le Goff, 1984) using metal pots as well as bells and rattles, was played to raise a great ruckus under the windows of old men married to young maidens when the greybeards refused to pay compensation for depriving the young people of the damsel in question. Here, the custom turns into torture. His face badly scratched, Don Quixote, usually quite tough, cries out in pain.

At that point, Altisidora, the duchess's cursed soul, enters the knight's room from the garden, to console him and treat him with St John's wort oil—sovereign healer of souls and bodies—while instilling guilt in his mind (Cassou, 1949, p. 854). Everything is his fault, and especially the fault of his squire, who refuses to be whipped. But Don Quixote resists the brainwashing and, eventually, during the five days when he must remain in bed, he escapes from his torturers, who are "greatly grieved at the unfortunate result of the joke". But again we wonder: is Don Quixote to be considered the victim of their sadistic scenarios?

Cervantes spares him such a fate, and shows that those who escape from such traps have in fact never been caught in them. They are the former children who have survived war, real or psychological, as is the case for Miss Rosa Coldfield, the old maid in William Faulkner's *Absalon, Absalon*, whom the author describes as being "contemporary with historical events" (1936, p. 52)—the Civil War. Another example is found in Tristram Shandy, in which the unfortunate hero is supported by his Uncle Toby, who is himself a wounded veteran (Sterne, 1999). In Robert Walser's *The Assistant* (1908), the despised handy man uncovers the abuse of a child in a highly respectable family. Here, Duena Rodriguez will prove to be a woman of the same calibre, and will help the knight reclaim his psyche.

The trauma market

As for Sancho, the agents of the duke attack his stomach, which is his "safe space", as Winnicott would say. The symposium over which he has to preside is held in a spacious chamber where "a table [is] laid out with royal magnificence" (De Cervantes, 1605/1615, p. 666).

Sancho is ushered in at the sound of clarions, and treated with great dignity. But Hunger is the real guest of honour at this feast. A haunting presence in the province of La Mancha in times of scarcity, it plays the starring role at this sham banquet. Although Sancho has "a laced bib" placed around his neck, he is condemned to fast.

The succulent dishes placed before him disappear one after the other, touched by the wand of the official physician, who declares them very harmful to his health. Accomplices of Molière's future Dr Purgon, the duke's spies are delighting in this torment of Tantalus inflicted on Sancho, and especially in the indignation with which he opposes medical authority.

Indeed, Sancho's diet, consisting largely of fatty foods, would horrify "healthy eaters". He is fond of "*ollas podridas* (and the rottener they are the better they smell, because [one] can put whatever [one] likes into them, so long as it is good to eat" (De Cervantes, 1605/1615, p. 681).

And since his love of food goes hand in hand with his love of free expression, woe to anyone who won't let him eat. The words fermenting in his stomach make him explode, "glowing all over with rage", against the bioethical propaganda attempting to control his appetite. Ready to "break [a chair] over [the] head" of the spoilsport, he is prepared to claim that he "served God in killing a bad doctor—a general executioner" (De Cervantes, 1605/1615, p. 668).

His hunger barely appeased after a frugal meal of bread and grapes, Sancho receives a message from the duke warning him that the island is threatened by imminent war. The lack of food and sleep—for he is deprived of his nap again—could push him to the brink of collapse, particularly since the case of the next plaintiff is particularly tragic.

A poor farmer, clearly as good as good bread, makes such a fine impression that the governor is ready to lean in his favour. A widower—for his pregnant wife was killed by a purge given by a bad doctor—he has two sons who are both students. He has come to request a grant for his younger son, who wants to set up house with his beloved. So far, so good. But then, the plaintiff makes the following portrait of the damsel: "She is so cleanly that not to soil her face she carries her nose turned up, as they say, so that one would fancy it was running away from her mouth; and with all this she looks extremely well, for she has a wide mouth; and but for wanting ten or a dozen teeth and grinders [...] I don't find her amiss" (De Cervantes, 1605/1615, p. 670).

So they must marry without having to live with the very wealthy parents of the girl, for fear that they discover that the farmer's son is epileptic, "possessed of the devil". Not at all impressed by the scoundrel's discourse—during which the majordomo made signs of encouragement, "for the rogue knew very well how to play his part"—Sancho refuses dryly any funds for the student, not mincing his words: "You whoreson rascal, you devil's own painter [...], six hundred ducats! [...] And why should I give them to you if I had them, you knave and blockhead?" (De Cervantes, 1605/1615, p. 671).

The action then commutes to the castle, for a veritable session of psychoanalysis between Don Quixote and Duena Rodriguez. As was the case in Cardenio's analysis, the madman of Sierra Morena (De Cervantes, 1605/1615, p.154), Cervantes' intention is to unmask perversion.

Madness checkpoint, in three scenes

When the reader is given a glimpse into Don Quixote's room, where he lies awake, "exceedingly moody and dejected, with his face [...] marked", so that he remained six days without appearing in public, the scene is that of a ceremonial play, at the moment when a spectre enters.

Scene 1: the uncanny

When he hears someone opening his door with a key, Don Quixote imagines that "the enamored damsel was coming to make an assault upon his chastity". He proffers at once a *vade retro* worthy of a terror-stricken virgin (De Cervantes, 1605/1615, p. 673). The following scene seems to come right out of an expressionist film made between the two world wars.

On one side, the knight is standing on his bed, looking like "the most extraordinary scarecrow that could be conceived", "wrapped from head to foot in a yellow satin coverlet, with a cap on his head, and his face and his moustaches tied up [...] to keep them from drooping and falling down", in Salvador Dalí style.

Facing him, he sees "a most venerable duena, in a long white bordered veil that covered and enveloped her from head to foot, [...] her eyes [...] covered by spectacles of great size, [advancing with noiseless steps, treading very softly, [holding] between the fingers of her left hand [...] a short lighted candle".

The collision between these two ghostly figures, both of them outsiders to the network of the ducal system, takes place in a timeless dimension where the phantoms of their respective stories hold a dominant place. The improbable transference that brings together these two "old children with white hair" (Lin Tsi, AD 867), as the Zen riddle says, frames two surviving images. Literally speaking. "from his watch-tower, [...] observing her costume and noting her silence, [...] he began crossing himself at a great rate", terrifying the white spectre which, with a "loud scream [...] let fall the candle in her fright, turned about to make off, but stumbling on her skirts [...] she measured her length with a mighty fall" (De Cervantes, 1605/1615, pp. 673–674).

Like in an analysis, when surreal images attempt to make contact with us, the analyst stumbles. Cervantes describes the event carefully, step by step. A syncopated rhythm, with a few steps forward and a few steps back, punctuated by screams, falls, and exclamations, sets the beat for the approach of a truth hitherto unspeakable. The dialogue of the two spectres begins in the dark.

The knight, "in his trepidation", knows from combat experience how to initiate contact instead of remaining petrified. Therefore, he starts by picking up the duena literally and figuratively. First, he uses words. "When faced with a vision, you must speak to make it move", as an Athapaskan Indian named Art Blue, speaking of his Vision Quest, told us in Manitoba. Saint Teresa of Avila gave the same advice to her nuns (Allendesalazar, 2001). The ceremonial formula must be pronounced at once: "I conjure thee, phantom, or whatever thou art, tell me what thou art and what thou wouldst with me?"

Indeed, his knightly services include, like those of a psychoanalyst dealing with madness or trauma, "doing good even to souls in purgatory".

The duena enters with a phantom hanging onto her. In fact, she is no less afraid than him, but her resistance to modernity allows her to display incredible sensitivity: "The unfortunate duena, hearing herself thus conjured, by her own fear guessed Don Quixote's."

Seeing his fear mirrored by this feminine double, at once terrified and gifted with prescience, Don Quixote can become conscious of his own unavowed fright. The two of them combine to form a plural body of survival, created by the fluctuation of their respective identities, in this early-version Sadian castle where they are uncertain of what they have become: Don Quixote has just been disfigured, and the duena is constantly humiliated. In fact, she is the only one who takes the knight's mission seriously: "Senor Don Quixote—if so be you are indeed Don Quixote—I am no phantom or specter or soul in purgatory [...], but Dona Rodriguez, duena of honor to my lady the duchess, and I come to you with one of those grievances your worship is wont to redress" (De Cervantes, 1605/1615, p. 674).

The double meaning at the unconscious level makes the knight suspicious. He interprets the "grievances" brought by the duena as sexual requests, customary at the castle: "Tell me, Senora Dona Rodriguez, [...] do you perchance come to transact any go-between, business. Because I must tell you I am not available for anybody's purpose, thanks to the peerless beauty of my lady Dulcinea del Toboso" (De Cervantes, 1605/1615, p. 674).

After conjuring the spectre of Celestina and her "seductive communications", Don Quixote agrees to discuss with her "all the commands you have […] and whatever you wish". The fundamental rule of free association is linked with sexual abstinence. As for the duena, she understands perfectly the reference to the infamous procuress, and protests. Not only is she not carrying anybody's messages, but, as she says, "I have a soul in my body still, and all my teeth"; and she adds: "I'm not far enough advanced in years to take to any such childish tricks."

In the name of this union of body and soul, which her masters were unable to destroy, she delivers a definitive judgement on the infantilisation taking place in that society.

Scene 2: casus belli

The analysis starts, but is stalled again by a negative attitude described with clinical precision. Going off to light her candle, Dona Rodriguez asks Don Quixote to wait for her, so that she can "lay [her] sorrows before [him]". Her transference is obvious when she refers to the knight as "one who relieves [the sorrows] of all the world". But, while she is gone, Don Quixote, although "tranquilly meditating", is assailed again by what has been unconsciously repressed: "Who knows but the devil, being wily and cunning, may be trying now to entrap me with a duena, having failed with empresses, queens, duchesses, marchionesses and countesses? Many a time have I heard it said […] that he will sooner offer you a flat-nosed wench than a roman-nosed one" (De Cervantes, 1605/1615, pp. 674–675).

To gain clarity, he conducts, as Freud did, a self-analysis of his own sexuality: "And who knows but this privacy, this opportunity, this silence, may awaken my sleeping desires?" In the end, he chooses to let desire stay repressed, and discovers the division of the subject by the unconscious: "But I must be out of my senses to think and utter such nonsense […]. In cases of this sort it is better to flee than to await the battle."

Projective defence mechanisms have been set in motion, of the type that trigger witch-hunts for less than this: "Is there a duena on earth that has fair flesh? Is there a duena in the world that escapes being ill-tempered, wrinkled and prudish? Avaunt, then, ye duena crew, undelightful to all mankind" (De Cervantes, 1605/1615, p. 675).

Before presenting their honest exchange, Cervantes has presented his characters as sexual beings. The reader discovers that Don Quixote is not made of stone in the presence of women, and that the duena is not as "undelightful" as her mistress makes her out to be.

Thus, the psychoanalytic encounter witnessed by the reader is unimaginable in the castle. It had never been planned for these two scarecrows to take the liberty of speaking to each other from behind their respective cracked mirrors. Indeed, both are survivors, both were betrayed by the ducal couple, and in this uncanny context of strange familiarity, they recognise each other as much more alive than the plaster figures around them.

During the second part of their encounter, another overlap of desires occurs. When the knight leaps out of bed to close the door and keep the repression of his fantasies safe, the duena is already back with a lighted candle. The phallus will not be denied! Her own projective identification as strong as his, she is as wary of his intentions as he is of hers, and she does not see it "as a sign of very great virtue that [he] should have got up out of bed". When he answers that he is as worried as she is, she promptly analyses the transference, understands that he is mistaking her for someone else, and delivers her second interpretation: "Of whom and against whom do you demand security, sir knight?" This allows unconscious desire to break through repression, and to be formulated by the knight in these words: "I am not marble, nor are you brass, nor is it now ten o'clock in the morning [...], and we are in a room [...] secluded and retired" (De Cervantes, 1605/1615, p. 675).

After these preliminary exchanges, Don Quixote goes on to analysis proper, offering the duena a gesture of therapeutic alliance: "But give me your hand, senora."

He assures her that she can count on his "protection [...], continence, and [...] sense of propriety"—commonly violated by dishonest therapists—and to seal his vow of good faith, "he kissed her right hand and took it in his own, she yielding it to him with equal ceremoniousness" (De Cervantes, 1605/1615, p. 675).

Thus, the ceremonial space opens with "a new loyalty", the term used by William Rivers, the British analyst of war trauma (Barker, 1992). The Furies can now enter time. In the margin, the Arab historian Cide Hamete Benengeli notes that "he would have given the best of the two tunics he had" to have witnessed this scene, as improbable as it was unexpected by the masters of the house.

Scene 3: anamnesis

To proceed with free association, Cardenio, the madman of the Sierre Morena, had lain down on the grass. This time, it is Don Quixote's turn to lie down again in his bed; he "wrapped his bedclothes round him and covered himself up completely, leaving nothing but his face visible". The duena "took her seat on a chair at some little distance", the knight was the first to break the silence, telling her: "Now […] you may unbosom yourself and out with everything you have in your sorrowful heart", for he was ready to listen. But should we conclude, from his supine position, that despite appearances and his offer to listen, she is the one acting as a *therapon* in Sancho's absence?

These two characters from bygone days have found a safe space, clearly removed from the torturers present in this violent place, where the duena can open her heart and Don Quixote can listen to her. Like in an analysis of trauma, she has forced her analyst to show his credentials and prove his reliability.

The case brought before the impartial knight is the story of a neglected child. Although she was born in a family descending from Asturian nobility—like everyone in the Austurias, as people used to say in jest at the time—she grew up without protection. Due to "the improvidence of my parents, who, I know not how, were unreasonably reduced to poverty", she was placed in the service of a countess at a very young age, since "for hemming and sewing [she has] never been surpassed by any".

Cervantes' critique of abandoning children to a fate of pseudo-autonomy is radical. After the death of her parents—which was not a great loss, since they took no interest in her—she was left in a precarious situation, "with nothing but the miserable wages and trifling presents that are given to servants of my sort in palaces" (De Cervantes, 1605/1615, p. 676). These protectors are no more reliable than those to whom young Cardenio had been entrusted. Courted by an esquire of the household, "a man somewhat advanced in years, full-bearded and personable, and above all as good as a gentleman as the king himself, for he came of a mountain stock"—the same jest as that concerning Asturians—she became his wife and gave birth to a daughter. And that is when her good fortune came to an end.

Mounted behind his squire on a mule, the countess lost her temper when he yielded the right of way on a narrow street, and struck him in the back with a bodkin, causing them both to fall to the ground. Wounded, the esquire became a laughing stock, "and it was chagrin at this […] that brought on his death". In other words, he died of post-traumatic stress disorder. For his wife, the post-traumatic flashbacks have remained vivid.

She needed to say no more. Don Quixote understood her clearly, after everything he had gone through himself. Betrayal of this kind, trivialised by those who witness it, makes time stop in its tracks. Remembering her husband's death, "she began to weep bitterly", and recounted how a second trauma had revived the painful wound. Their daughter had been seduced and abandoned by the son of a very wealthy farmer who "lends [the duke] money, and is constantly going security for his debts" (De Cervantes, 1605/1615, p. 678). Once again, the abuse is shrouded in silence, and the duena asks for redress.

Without a doubt, Don Quixote is the right man for the job. In the first novel, he demonstrated repeatedly that in addition to defending widows and maidens "as virginal as the mothers who bore them", the inscription of paternal traumas is his speciality. He understands that, beyond what was done to the daughter, the reparation concerns the humiliation suffered by her father, who wanders like the lost soul of one who was the victim of a wrongful death never avenged. And no wonder! Before the knight can utter a word, the duena insists on informing him of the corruption reigning in the household, where "all is not gold that glitters" (De Cervantes, 1605/1615, p. 678).

The rotting away of the social link often takes the appearance of eternal youth founded on the denial of death, which spreads a foul odour just the same. First, through the fetid breath of the pretentious Altisidora, the furious duena tells Don Quixote, and above all through the evil humours "of which [the duchess] is full", and which are evacuated by means of two drains she has, one in each leg, under her skirts. It is not a pretty sight, what one sees under the skirts of the powers that be, especially when it concerns the secrets of eternal youth, which in Cervantes' time had become Countess Bathory's speciality.

Suddenly alarmed, the duena becomes aware—but too late—that "the walls have ears". Before Don Quixote can react, someone lifts her skirts in the dark, for in her fright she dropped the candle again. Invisible, silent beings have seized her by the throat, so that for half an hour she can be given a beating, which the knight does not escape either: "they pinched him so fast and so hard that he was driven to defend himself with his fists, and all this in marvellous silence" (De Cervantes, 1605/1615, p. 678).

After the trashing by the castle's security service, the protagonists go their separate ways without another word, leaving the duena's grievances in suspense after this incredible session. They have been able to wrest an intense episode of spiritual exchange from the shenanigans of pleasures and desires, to impose the analysis of a trauma condemned to non-existence.

The duena spoke without interruption for over two consecutive pages to a "passionate witness", as formulated by Dori Laub, a witness who "has been there experientially, and who waits with patience and with readiness for [the other] to join him" (Laub, 1992, p. 69). Don Quixote was able to listen and to hear the duena's story as resonances of his adventures in the first novel, thanks to an extraordinary transference the brutes brutally attempt to silence.

In this silence, "Sancho claims our attention" in counterpoint, to play his melodic line during a reprieve in the reign of terror that will come down on him as well.

Night watch

The squire sends Don Quixote a message to sum up his position. He lets the knight know that "he …, fool, boor, and clown as he was, held his own against them all …, without giving up a right or taking a bribe" (De Cervantes, 1605/1615, pp. 680–681).

The reader knows Sancho's political philosophy, based on equality before death: "when God sends the dawn, he sends it for all". But, for all that, he does not renounce his authority: "Make yourself honey and the flies eat you" (De Cervantes, 1605/1615, p. 681).

Incredibly, the fat slob disfigured by Avellaneda surprises the duke's henchmen, and particularly the young majordomo, who remarks: "I am filled with wonder when I see a man like your worship, entirely without learning (for I believe you have none at all) say such things, and so full of sound maxims and sage remarks, very different from what was expected of your worship's intelligence by those who sent us …" (De Cervantes, 1605/1615, p. 681).

He praises Sancho's intelligence, just when the governor decides to make night rounds, "to purge this island of all manner of uncleanness and of all idle good-for-nothing vagabonds, for I would have you know that lazy idlers are the same thing in a State as the drones in a hive, that eat up the honey the industrious bees make".

A word to the wise! Sancho the beekeeper has had occasion to observe that in early fall the bees kill the males, so that only the queen and the worker bees remain clustered in the hive during the winter season.

But we now know that male bees are also useful to the republic because they ventilate the hive when the weather is warm, to keep the temperature constant. But we needn't dwell on this here. The social organisation of bees has been a topic in political science since antiquity.

The reference here is to Book 4 of Virgil's *The Georgics*, in which the poet pays homage to the old veteran of Taranto (c. 29 BC, lines 114–148) who keeps bees on his little parcel of land, and to the bees' system of government as a model republic. Virgil's own father, a beekeeper near Mantua, lost his property when a new law granted confiscated land to Roman army veterans. The pastoral setting allows Sancho to condemn, along with male bees, the state's freeloading, when it depletes the public purse to put on shows for idle minds—the daily routine at the ducal castle. The majordomo understands that, somehow or other, Sancho has subverted the system: "Every day we see something new in the world; jokes become realities, and the jokers find the tables turned upon them" (De Cervantes, 1605/1615, p. 681).

Indeed, the duchess will soon show herself to be a vacuous ninny full of prejudices. As a matter of fact, Don Quixote and Sancho do not expect much of institutions. They know that the effects of truth revealed by their actions will not last. Everyone agrees that Sancho's government is exemplary, yet there will be no crowds of demonstrators shouting "Sancho for president!" Similarly, the revolt of the duena who allied herself with Don Quixote proves to be short-lived.

The governor will encounter this passion around the corner in the shape of a young man, like in the Homeric era of Greek gods. The *Night Watch* immortalised by Rembrandt, starts out well, allowing Sancho to put his plan into action. In the midst of "a fair-sized squadron" of alguacils and notaries, he marches with his governor's staff through the streets of the town (De Cervantes, 1605/1615, p. 681). An old French song describes the situation:

> Who goes there so late, companions of the Marjolaine,
> Who goes there so late, fording the riverbed?
> It's the knight watch, companions of the Marjolaine ….
> And what does the knight seek? A maiden to wed.

Such night-time rituals are still practised in Guanajuato, Mexico, a traditional site of Cervantian culture. During the *callejoneada* (walking serenade), students dressed in black cape and doublet trimmed with ribbons stroll the streets in small groups, playing guitar and singing satirical verses, accompanied by young boys, like the young announcer of Master Pedro's puppet show, who recite burlesque poetry.

This is how Sancho walks through the streets, proud of himself, "quite a sight to see!" The noise of swords clashing stops the procession.

First station: at the exit of a gambling den

Where the duena's revelations about the corruption of grandees are confirmed.

The case brought before Sancho concerns a quarrel over cheating at gambling. The false witness charged with attesting that the game is not rigged has not received his part of the gain. This quarrel is settled by the governor, who orders the first of man to give his accomplice the money owed, the second man to be expelled from the island, and both of them to pay a fine for the benefit of the poor in prisons. Sancho is not joking: "I'll hang you on a gibbet, or at least the hangman will by my orders; not a word from either of you, or I'll make him feel my hand" (De Cervantes, 1605/1615, p. 682).

A notary enlightens Sancho about the identity of the gambling house *padrino*: "This one at least, your worship will not be able to get rid of, for a great man owns it, and what he loses every year is beyond all comparison more than what he makes by the cards. [...] and as the vice of gambling has become common, it is better that men should play in houses of repute [where] notorious sharpers dare not attempt to play their tricks." The protection of gambling "lords" is preferable by far to what goes on in places "where they catch an unlucky fellow in the small hours of the morning and skin him alive" (De Cervantes, 1605/1615, p. 683).

Each era has its addictions, which promote "the complicity of the elite with organised crime", denounced by Hannah Arendt in *The Origins of Totalitarianism* (1951). How are we to avoid this? Cervantes offers the worried reader an answer in the next section, where medieval "gay science" is regenerated.

Second station: dealing with a fugitive

A youth is brought before Sancho, who "as soon as he saw the officers of justice [...] ran like a deer, a sure proof that he must be some evil-doer".

He is to escape, as Cervantes did at the same age, when he fled to Italy after being accused of wounding a master mason in a duel. Caught by the officer, the youth has no choice but to speak in his own defence. During his questioning, his witty retorts leave Sancho speechless. Not one to be tongue-tied as a rule, the squire finds his freedom of expression hampered by his position of authority. As the fast-paced exchange unfolds, the reader witnesses the production of freedom in a desperate situation. The governor first adopts a paternal attitude: "What did you run for, fellow?"

Quick as a flash, the youth challenges his condescending tone: "it was to avoid answering all the questions officers of justice put".

Sancho then goes on to routine questions:

> "What are you by trade?"
> "A weaver."
> "And what do you weave?"
> "Lance heads, [...]."

The boy makes Sancho lose his good humour and forces him into the role of a cop:

> "You're facetious with me! You plume yourself on being a wag? Very good; and where were you going just now?"
> "To take the air, senor."
> Back to a routine question again: "And where does one take the air in the island?"
> "Where it blows."
>
> (De Cervantes, 1605/1615, p. 684)

The image created has taken on an unexpected meaning. The air one takes when strolling becomes the air rushing into the sails of a boat, or the air propelling a kite, which is not so easy to catch. Burdened by his official function, which inhibits him from using his proverbs freely, Sancho wants to break this insolence and its word games: "you are a smart youth; but take notice that I am the air, and that I blow upon you a-stern, and send you to gaol".

The sarcastic tone takes the poetry out of the metaphor, reminding us of the chaplain in chapter I, who caused the student to be locked away for good (De Cervantes, 1605/1615, p. 401). Sancho uses the same type of rhetoric. He turns the victim's words against him and stifles him by refusing the breathing space of a dialogue. "Ho there! Lay hold of him and take him off; I'll make him sleep there tonight without air."

But contrary to the licentiate, the young man has not been subdued by years of hospitalisation. For the third time, he refuses to comply: "By God, your worship will make me sleep in gaol just as soon as make me king."

Sancho doesn't understand. His questions transfer the advantage to the youth, who turns them into riddles: "Why shan't I [...]? Have I not the power to arrest thee and release thee whenever I like?" As long as the dialogue continues, the boy can fight and break free with words: "All the power your worship has, won't be able to make me sleep in gaol." Sancho is exasperated, and starts to talk about chains, irons, and all the rest, with no effect on the accused: "That's ridiculous, the fact is, all the men on earth will not make me sleep in prison" (De Cervantes, 1605/1615, p. 401).

Suspicion of sorcery and the stakes of the Inquisition are conjured up: "Tell me, you devil, have you got any angel that will deliver you, and take off the irons I am going to order them to put upon you?" But another sort of magic springs forth, that of poetry: "if I don't choose to sleep, and choose to remain awake all night without closing an eye, will your worship with all your power be able to make me sleep if I don't choose?" (De Cervantes, 1605/1615, p. 704).

Disarmed by the stubbornness of the child who, from the time he is born, can refuse to close an eye and can resist all lullabies, pleas, and other forms of bribery, the tyrant-to-be gives in. Fortunately, this governor is not the kind of pervert who nips in the bud any attempt at existing outside his sphere of influence.

Out of the jousting, a free subject is produced. The scheme—for such it clearly was—which had aimed at turning Sancho into a common torturer, failed. Sancho loves life and recognises that he is dealing with a wizard of language, full of vitality, a Green Man with leaves and flowers sprouting from his mouth, who can quell all night-time fears. Therefore, he makes peace with the elfin character who has brought him back to himself, just as the duena had restored the knight's soul: "Well then, go, and God be with you, be off home to sleep, and God give you sound sleep, for I don't want to rob you of it." He even analyses the tyrannical transference into which he almost fell: "but for the future, [...] don't joke with the authorities, because you may come across someone who will bring down the joke on your own skull".

By contrast, the two young people the reader will meet subsequently are not of the same calibre. Cervantes wants to prevent the reader from falling into the stereotyped idealisation of youth.

Third station: disguised children

The Green Man's genius is not given to anyone; every attempt to escape is unique. After the breath of fresh air provided by Cervantes' youth, two adolescents, brother and sister, are brought before the governor in turn; this case was not part of the Duke's pre-planned programme. They had traded clothes. Their transgression was motivated by the desire to escape one night in secret from their overprotective milieu, to see the world. They are very touching, and the girl is fascinating in her tearful innocence. But she ends up irritating Sancho, for her desires are limited to seeing bullfights, javelin games, and theatre performances, equivalent to today's movies and rave parties.

Tired of the girl's whining, Sancho daydreams about marrying his daughter Sanchica to her brother. In the meantime, he loses no time sending them back home: "this has been a very childish affair, and to explain your folly and rashness there was no necessity for all this delay and these tears and sighs" (De Cervantes, 1605/1615, p. 687).

Cervantes depicts their infantilisation as diametrically opposed to the boy's desire to get away from the suffocating atmosphere of a society which, after discovering the New World, gradually closes in on itself.

Homefront

In the meantime, Cide Hamete, the Arab historian and "painstaking investigator of the minute points of this veracious history" (De Cervantes, 1605/1615, p. 687), has enquired about the masked assailants who aggressed the duena and the knight. What Hamete found out is that, informed by another duena, the duchess and her protégée Altisidora listened outside Don Quixote's door, until the unbearable revelations of Altisidora's foul breath and the duchess's drains drove them to action, "for indignities offered to their charms and self esteem mightily provoke the anger of women and make them eager for revenge" (De Cervantes, 1605/1615, p. 689).

A vendetta was organised against Sancho's family, on the theme: "Some day my prince will come ..." The duchess wants to persuade Sancho's wife that her dreams will come true thanks to her. In passing, she will rehabilitate her own image damaged by Duena Rodriguez, by presenting herself to simple folk as a television celebrity who deigns to bring them into the limelight with her for a few minutes.

Who would not be ecstatic? Teresa Panza certainly was!

Entry into the sphere of the pastoral is accomplished through a page on horseback. He spotted "a young girl [...] who seemed to be about fourteen", washing clothes on the riverbank. Barefoot, jaunty, and light, Sanchica takes the page to her mother in the village, "skipping, running, and capering, [...] her hair hanging about her", all excited that a smart-looking gentleman is bringing news of her father. Barely younger than Altisidora, her spontaneity contrasts with the affected airs put on by the duchess's protégées or Celestina's "girls".

Teresa also offered a complete contrast. "She was not very old, though plainly past forty", and had no time to worry about her age or appearance. She stood before the page, "strong, healthy, vigorous, and sundried" (De Cervantes, 1605/1615, p. 690), and she saw coming a mile away the smooth-talker who addresses her as "the lawful and only wife of [a] rightful governor". With a well-placed "Ah, senor, get up", which reminds me of my grandmother, she refuses to have her hands kissed.

Not discouraged in the least, the page submits proof of the miracle; he takes out of his pocket "a string of coral beads with gold clasps", finer than the trinkets usually given to the native women. And that was not all! After placing the beads around her neck, he shows her the letters from Sancho and from the duchess, whose fabulous plan is to make Teresa and her daughter stars *ex nihilo*.

"[L]ost in astonishment and her daughter just as much" (De Cervantes, 1605/1615, p. 690), Teresa sets aside the suspicions she expressed in her recent quarrel with her husband. It must be said that in the letter the page reads her, the duchess addresses her as if they were on equal footing. The great lady speaks to her as she would to a friend. To reinforce the impression of their closeness, she claims reciprocity and asks her to send a dozen acorns from her village in exchange for the golden beads. The duchess is portrayed as the perfect patroness. "Ah, what a good, plain, lowly lady!" said Teresa, "and not [like] the gentlewomen we have in this town, that [...] go to church with as much airs as if they were queens, no less, and seem to think they are disgraced if they look at a farmer's wife!" (De Cervantes, 1605/1615, p. 691).

And she went out onto the street thrumming the letters and capering in front of the curate and Sanson Carrasco, who just happened to come by. She was now ready to marry off Sanchica to any philanderer, provided he was as rich as the duchess promised, and that she and Sanchica would be seen together in a handsome carriage, dressed in their finery, to the envy of all the neighbourhood women. Sanchica, clearly her mother's daughter, demands half the necklace for herself. Despite her hyper-excitement—hypomania, as the experts would say—Teresa acts in sharp contrast to ducal self-centredness: "It is all for thee, my child [...], but let me wear it round my neck for a few days, for verily it seems to make my heart glad."

And the daughter, in turn, naively reveals her oedipal wish to see her round-bellied father "wear trunk hose", and be puffed up by the tabloids, with their stories of the "successful", the "royal", and the "ducal", movie stars and fashion moguls, sports and media celebrities. Amazed by the hymn of glory sung by Teresa and Sanchica to the rhythm of a multitude of proverbs—as if, the curate says: "all this family of the Panzas are born with a sackful of proverbs in their insides" (De Cervantes, 1605/1615, p. 694)—the barber/curate/Carrasco trio cannot believe their eyes. But the evidence is there, attesting that the Quixotic delusion has become reality.

Certain details—that the island is not on the seashore, for instance, make the student suspicious—"*dubitat Augustinus*", he says in Latin—and he believes all this "to be something in the line of [...] enchantment" (De Cervantes, 1605/1615, p. 694). But the page gives nothing away; instead, he agrees to share a meal with the curate, who invites him to "come and do penance with me". So he will not enjoy the delicious omelette with bacon prepared for him by Sanchica on her mother's orders, to "give him his dinner like a prince". One mustn't get one's values mixed up.

And yet, the duchess's plan to make short work of the young girl fails at the last moment. Something resists in the Panzas' space of safety, which the duchess is unable to seize. The members of this family are not so dumb, nor so vulnerable, as to be taken in by her mumbo jumbo. Aloof to flattery and false promises, they draw their strength from the oral tradition Sanchica handles brilliantly, in the style of self-mockery. Describing herself as one who "goes stretched at her ease [...] as if she was a she-pope", she imagines herself seated in a coach with her mother, defying the gossip: "See that rubbish, that garlic-stuffed fellow's daughter ..." And she is thrilled to think of the gasps of bystanders: "But let them trump through the mud, and let me go in my coach with my feet off the ground" (De Cervantes, 1605/1615, p. 694).

And she plays up to the page in "handsome apparel": "take me with you, senor, behind you on your horse [...], what a dainty lass you must take me for!" Teresa stops her at once: "Hush, girl, [...] you don't know what you're talking about." The page understands how things stand. He can't do as he pleases with Sanchica: "Senora Teresa says more than she is aware of" (De Cervantes, 1605/1615, p. 695).

As long as everyone does his job, all will be well. Teresa knows how to be a mother and gains the respect of the boy who is used to the rakish ways of the castle.

Teresa's letters to Sancho and to the duchess will be received two chapters further. To escape Carrasco's control, she has them written by a young penman in exchange for "a cake and a couple of eggs". Decidedly, the Panzas are able to protect their freedom of thinking and of speech. But Teresa would betray her name if, in the letter to her husband, she did not confess her ecstasy—equal to that of the Saint of Avila: "I promise thee and swear as a Catholic Christian that I was within two fingers' breath of going mad I was so happy. [...] I thought I should have dropped dead with pure joy; and thou knowest they say sudden joy kills as well as great sorrow." The clinical signs of a state of trance are clearly present: "Sanchica, thy daughter, [...] leaked from sheer happiness" (De Cervantes, 1605/1615, pp. 706–707).

Like the other Teresa, who could abandon herself to mystical raptures and yet founded over thirty Carmels while providing psychotherapy to her nuns, Teresa does not neglect earthly realities, and gives Sancho news of everyday life in the village. So-and-so's son has received the first orders, the daughter of so-and-so says she is pregnant by him, the olive harvest was ruined by draught, lightning struck the gibbet, a company of soldiers took away three of the village girls, whose names must not be mentioned in case they come back.

In France, they still remember—hush!—in the countryside where my grandmother lived, the girls who left for America with their soldiers, after the First World War, and who came back disappointed. All these details, laughable in the eyes of the ducal court, are valuable landmarks of memory for the village-dwellers.

Teresa's letter to the duchess shows that she is keenly aware of the lady's need to impress. Therefore, she promises the "lady of my soul, to [...] go to Court to stretch myself at ease in a coach, and make all those I have envying me already burst their eyes out" (De Cervantes, 1605/1615, p. 706). But when the letter ends, the unconscious reveals itself when Teresa addresses her so-called new friend as "your high mightiness".

Logical impasse

Reassured, albeit with some delay, about the reliability of his "homefront"—as the British call the women left at home while they are away at war—Sancho can fight the war against the enemies who try to destroy him. Deprived of his master, of food, and of rest, he is confronted with new cases early the next morning, without having had any breakfast. Here, Cervantes shows how to transform a session of mind control worthy of a Lao Dai into verbal sparring as it was practised by the Chan master Lin Tsi (AD 867) in China, in the eleventh century.

The riddle submitted to the governor by the stranger who is the first case of the day resembles one of his "Dialogues between the Host and the Visitor". Lin Tsi poses an enigma to the visitor, who is beaten if he cannot solve it. Conversely, if he is able to answer, the latter pulls the master out of his chair. One would think the spiritual exercises of oriental monasticism had been introduced into the monasteries frequented by Cervantes.

As we watch, like in a Zen painting drawn in Indian ink and wash tint, we see a powerful river and a bridge; at the end of the bridge, one can see the rope of a gallows. In those days, there was no fooling around with logic. The paradox presented to Sancho takes the form of an enigma resembling that of Epimenides, the famous Cretan who declares that all Cretans are liars. Is he telling the truth?

The toll to pay to cross the bridge is to state under oath, before four judges, where one is going and to what purpose. Lies are punishable by hanging. Along comes a joker who swears that his purpose is to hang on these gallows. Consulted by one of the toll judges, Sancho must decide on the spot what to do with this traveller: "If we let this man pass free he has sworn falsely, and by the law he ought to die; but if we hang him, as he swore he was going to die on this gallows, and therefore swore the truth, by the same law he ought to go free" (De Cervantes, 1605/1615, p. 697).

The man's life is at stake. "Answer, answer quickly", the masters of the "sudden response" in the Chan tradition used to say.

But Sancho takes time to think, asks to hear the question again, and then delivers his judgement promptly: the man should be "divided into two parts". Evidently, binary abstract reasoning can be lethal.

Instead of this sinister solution, Sancho's next proposal is reminiscent of another Zen dialogue (Izutsu, 2001), in which a young illiterate servant in a monastery overturns a jug with his foot, in response to the question "what does this thing mean?" As a result, he is praised by his master for overthrowing the endless debates of the learned. This famous story illustrates Wittgenstein's formula: "the sign [has] meaning even when its bearer ceases to exist" (1953, Aphorism 41), which becomes in Lacanian terms: "the word is the murder of the thing" (Lacan, 2007). Similarly, Sancho has overturned the logical impasse, and has emerged as a subject of speech, instead of remaining the object of ducal sadism: "as the arguments for condemning him and for absolving him are exactly balanced, they should let him pass freely, as it is always more praiseworthy to do good than to do evil; this I would give signed with my name if I knew how to sign" (De Cervantes, 1605/1615, p. 697).

Drawing from Ancient Indian tradition, Louis Renou relates other examples of sharp-witted jousting, in which the solution to the enigma subverts binary ways of thinking. The aim, writes the Sanskrit scholar, is to reset in motion time stuck in amorphous duration, "when the era is in confusion", and to allow the "embryo bearing the weight of the world" to develop—a precept Sancho and his master defend above all else (Renou, 1972).

The perilous bridge of language

Governor Sancho has changed the rules of the game by engaging his word and his reputation, backed up by that of his master, to loyalties stronger than the mesh of the net that is tightening around them. In order to escape a flattened, two-dimensional world, he has only to invoke Don Quixote, a third party with a cracked helmet, all the more efficient since he is physically absent: "what I have said in this case is not out of my own head, but one of the many precepts my master Don Quixote gave me the night before I left to become governor of this island, [...] and it was this, that when there was any doubt about the justice of a case, I should lean to mercy" (De Cervantes, 1605/1615, p. 697).

Although he lost the piece of paper bearing his master's advice, the precepts are inscribed in his memory and come into his mind when he needs them. They are called up by a transference having less to do with abstract debate than with saving someone's life. Thus, the oral tradition allows the inscription of unwritten laws which, in an emergency, saves the life of the mind.

Sancho's judgement is similar to that of Solomon. But in this perilous passage, the story evokes the tradition of bridge-building. In far-off times, a human sacrifice was demanded to appease the river god, and the victim's bones were integrated into the pillars of the bridge.

Cervantes advises the reader, if he wants to cross the perilous bridge of speech, to give up paralysing sophisms and, above all, let go of the burden of vanity. Then, his light psyche will be able to cross confidently, knowing that the invisible pillar on the other side, on the side of the Other, will hold.

Henceforth, Governor Sancho is in the process of winning the psychological war with the people at the court who had seen him as a dummy. Ready to cross over to his side, the majordomo disobeys the injunction to starve him, and orders a hearty meal for him. Soon, news arrive that Teresa, contrary to the duena's irresponsible parents, has not allowed her daughter to leave home. Reassured about his homefront, Sancho can also count on his master who, from his headquarters at the castle, writes to him that his political conduct is well founded, and sends him more useful precepts at the same time.

He recommends humility, but not too much; elegance, but without coquetry, abundant provisions to avoid hunger; few laws, but observed; to be "a father to virtue and a stepfather to vice, [and] not always strict, not yet always lenient" (De Cervantes, 1605/1615, p. 699); to "visit prisons, but also markets, since not all thieves are locked up; resist addiction in all its forms: to money, to gambling, to wine, to drugs, to women"—through which "those that have dealings with thee [...] will bring their batteries to bear upon thee [...], till they have brought thee down to the depths of perdition" (De Cervantes, 1605/1615, p. 699).

Like a good general, Don Quixote informs his man of the page's visit to Teresa, and asks him to clarify the identity of the majordomo who so closely resembles Señora Trifaldi. Then, without warning, the knight frees his squire of any obligation of allegiance, disclosing his unexpected decision "of giving over very shortly this idle life I am now leading, for

I was not born for it". He then alludes to something that "will put me out of favour with the duke and duchess".

The reader can anticipate the events that will overturn the scheduled entertainment programme at the castle. Although he is "sorry for it", the knight will follow his desire, "for after all I must obey my calling rather than their pleasure".

In his answer to this letter, Sancho objects that it is not the right time to change plans. Proud of his success, he sends his master a brilliant report on his good government. Contrary to others, he has not been idle, nor has he worked for personal profit. He carried out quality controls on the markets, and protested against dietary fanaticism which kills patients by starving them.

"The Constitutions of Sancho Panza", a historical document, will testify to the creation of "an *alguacil* of the poor", who will separate the genuine poor from the fake beggars, "for many a sturdy thief or drunkard goes about under cover of a makebelieve crippled limb or a sham sore" (De Cervantes, 1605/1615, p. 702).

Yet, despite his shrewdness, Sancho does not perceive the war brewing on the borders of the little world he believes he governs so well. This war breaks out both on his island and at the castle. At the same time, like in a musical counterpoint, "two women [...] draped in mourning from head to foot" (De Cervantes, 1605/1615, p. 703) burst through the castle door and throw themselves at the knight's feet.

The art of the fugue

In *The Purple Rose of Cairo* (Allen, 1985), the characters step off the screen and enter the movie theatre. Similarly, the two women have broken the mirror of the ducal performances by an unforeseeable act, since they have an authentic request of real wrongs to right. Of course, the reader has recognised Dona Rodriguez and her daughter, whose mourning garb exhibits the presence of the paternal ghost. Like Hamlet's father, he comes back to ask, through them, reparation for the felony that caused his death and deceived his daughter. Perverts can only be caught by surprise.

When Dona Rodriguez lifts her veil, the bearded matron's superproduction turns into harsh reality. The words and gestures are the same, but a tone of sincerity throws the ducal comedy off pitch. Without looking at her masters, she "[turned] to Don Quixote and [addressed] herself to him". Evidently, she was not intimidated by the beating; the transference created between the two of them during the night remained solid. The ducal couple is at a loss, "for though they thought her a simpleton and a weak creature, they did not think her capable of crazy pranks" (De Cervantes, 1605/1615, p. 703).

The duena's craziness consists in having found her *therapon*, her second in combat.

This simpleton pushover suddenly displays soldierly resources and revives expressions emptied of sense by her masters, wrongs to be redressed, and honour to be defended.

Around 1600, Hamlet used actors to enact the murder of his father before his assassins. Similarly, the duena reveals publicly the mistreatment inflicted on her, before those who inflicted it. It is no longer possible to consider normal—but everyone does it!—that the murderous uncle married his victim's wife, that the duena's husband was stubbed in the back by his mistress, and that her sixteen-year-old daughter was seduced by one of the duke's protégés. Cervantes, a contemporary of Shakespeare who died the same week he did, also used theatre within theatre to "demonstrate" monsters, and to speak openly of a pervert "wrong-doer" and of "malfeasance" (De Cervantes, 1605/1615, p. 704), old-fashioned words that ward off denial.

Just as Hamlet draws from the vision of his father's ghost the energy needed to unmask the criminal, Dona Rodriguez has found, in her session with Don Quixote, the strength to speak of the vile death of her daughter's father. She addresses him now directly, because he had listened to her "some days since" when she "gave [him] an account of the injustice and treachery of a wicked farmer to my dearly beloved daughter", giving her the courage to break the silence. And she adds: "for to expect that my lord the duke will do me justice is to ask pears from the elm tree, for the reason I stated privately to your worship" (De Cervantes, 1605/1615, p. 704).

Don Quixote understands the political stakes. After his usual formula promising "to obtain redress" for the injury done to the maiden, he specifies that it is "the chief object of [his] profession [...] to destroy the oppressors" (De Cervantes, 1605/1615, p. 704). Words that were to resonate in future centuries! But this time, the knight does not attack the castle. He simply puts the duke in his place, the place of an abuser who thought he was above the law. The subversive paradigm is still that of the Sotties, in which the jesters, led by Mother Folly, take away the tyrant's official garb, to reveal to the public a fool's costume hidden under his solemn appearance, covering up his crazy passion for power, which perpetuates perversion.

Forced to play the game, the duke "accepted the challenge" and picked up the glove thrown in the middle of the hall by Don Quixote, "in the name of his vassal, [for] breaking faith with this poor damsel, who was a maiden and now by his misdeed is none" (De Cervantes, 1605/1615, p. 704). The duel in a jousting arena is to take place six days later, in the courtyard of the castle, with the customary arms, "without trickery, guile, or charms of any sort".

The challenge seems exaggerated today, when virginity is not such a prized asset. Moreover, the girl herself is tired of being exhibited and scolded by Don Quixote for her readiness "to believe lovers' promises". She is probably thinking that without these two clowns, she would have handled things differently. But in her era, "all in tears and covered with shame and confusion", she had to obey her mother, without really understanding that through her, in fact, reparation was enacted for the crime which left her without a father at birth. Oftentimes, in the course of an analysis of repressed desires, there suddenly emerges a traumatic scene in which phantoms of the lineage demand justice.

Teresa's letters arrive just in time to provide some tension relief. Now that the duke is losing his authority, the letter to the duchess aptly bears the heading: "Letter for my lady the Duchess So-and-So, of I don't know where" (De Cervantes, 1605/1615, p. 705). The public reading of the letter transforms the peasant woman into an object of mockery, diverting the focus from the disgrace revealed by the two plaintiffs.

In fact, the duchess has promptly had them expelled from her service. Treated like outsiders, they have no other protectors than the knight, whose value on the stock market of that era was no higher than that of the damsel's virginity. Both women are ejected into the limitless space of hate that perverts generate when they are unmasked. Here, Cervantes makes us aware of the length of time it takes to regain freedom.

A word to the wise! Back from the village, the page has brought the duchess the cheese Teresa sent her as a gift, because it was "particularly good and superior to those of Tronchon" (De Cervantes, 1605/1615, p. 708). But the duchess does not care. She knows nothing of the symbolism of "The fool holding a cheese", seen in medieval illuminated manuscripts. Entirely absorbed by the immediate consumption of the life of others, she is not interested in cheeses, whose maturing, says

Hildegarde von Bingen, like soul maturation, takes time and may become corrupted.

Thrust!

Time is a major character in the second *Don Quixote*. Now, the knight's life, like that of Cervantes, is nearing its end. To remind us that the cyclical time of nature makes the wheel of fortune turn, Cervantes quotes Cide Hamete, "the Mahometan philosopher", who now speaks "of the rapidity with which Sancho's government came to an end, melted away, disappeared, vanished as it were in smoke and shadow" (De Cervantes, 1605/1615, p. 709).

In that century of Baroque art and religious wars, La Boétie, Montaigne's friend, uses the same metaphor to depict the futility of a people's efforts to feed the constant greed of tyrants. The latter's unquenchable thirst consumes everyone else's energy, reducing it to ashes (La Boétie, 1548). Those who exhaust themselves supporting them, helping them, and even bringing about changes and reforms, as Sancho did, are thrown away after use. Cervantes resorts to using biblical allusions to illustrate this.

In the middle of the seventh night, after having finally eaten and drunk as much as he wanted, the governor can enjoy some well-earned rest, now that his task is accomplished. But instead, he is shaken up violently by the manoeuvres of the political system which he consented to serve so well. Bedlam breaks out, with bells, drums, trumpets, and frightened cries, while he sleeps: "To arms, to arms, [...]! The enemy is in the island [...] and we are lost" (De Cervantes, 1605/1615, p. 709).

Naked swords and lighted torches suggest that the enemy is at the door. In fact, a manhunt has begun, targeting the governor in "his shirt" (De Cervantes, 1605/1615, p. 710), who was easy prey. The need to arm him serves as a pretext to immobilise him between two shields: "he was walled and borded up [...] and unable to bend his knees or stir a single step". As soon as he tried to advance, he "fell to the ground with such a crash that he fancied he had broken himself all to pieces [...] like a tortoise enclosed in its shell, or a side of bacon between two kneading troughs, or a boat bottom up on the beach" (De Cervantes, 1605/1615, p. 710).

Or like a cockroach on its back, akin to Gregor Samsa, the hero of Kafka's *Metamorphosis* (1915), another man sacrificed to his parasitic, whining family. His father is jobless, his mother a hypochondriac, his sister a would-be artist; Gregor, a travelling salesman, is their only provider: "Over the long years, [his parents] had developed the conviction that Gregor was set up for life in his firm and, in addition, they had so much to do nowadays with their present troubles that all foresight was foreign to them."

The family system enslaves a child for the physical and psychological well-being of his relatives: "They had become quite accustomed to it, both the family and Gregor as well. They took the money with thanks, and he happily surrendered it, but the special warmth was no longer present." Until the day when Gregor finally dares to admit to himself that he is tired of carrying this weight, when his back rigidifies—like that of Sancho turned into a turtle—and he finds he is an insect laying on his "armour-hard back", with only his thin arms and legs extending from it. Some fifty pages later, after the death of the tyrannised child, the monstruous insect he had become in the eyes of the family is mercilessly thrown in the trash.

All is well that ends well! The family is regenerated by this trifling human sacrifice. In case the reader might be horrified by this assassination, Kafka ruthlessly demonstrates that murderers of the psyche act without remorse, for their future is secure: "Leaning back comfortably in their seats, they talked to each other about future prospects [...], for the three of them had employment [...] which was extremely favourable and with especially promising prospects."

The two heroes are threatened by the same fate: to be sacrificed in order to renew their hosts' energy.

Time regained

The manhunt is a regular passtime of tyrannical systems, be it in a household, at school, at work, or on the street, whatever the age of the bullied victim and the slogans of his persecutors. Completely isolated and deprived of his transferential apparatus—his master, the ass, and Teresa, whose letter has not yet reached him—Sancho serves as a human shield sent to the slaughter by the jubilant mob. Among the terrifying acts to which he is subjected there is the stage trick of the woman "sawed in half", except that in his case the box has no false bottom. Struck by sword blows, trampled by some, crushed by others, "he [...] gathered himself together and made himself small [in] that narrow compass [...] sweating and sweating again ...".

Cervantes had been well acquainted with torture in the bagnios of Algiers, where it was a daily occurrence. In case we ever have to endure such a torment, he provides us with a guide outlining its stages and the steps to possible escape.

First, there is the impression of imminent death, exacerbated to the point where one wishes, like Sancho, to see oneself dead. Then comes the unexpected reanimation, to cries of "Victory, victory!" intended to produce a feeling of exaggerated gratitude towards the "friends" who, after the agony, bring one back to life. Finally, the torturers may become worried when, despite the vigilance of doctors, psychiatrists, and psychologists, their victim remains in danger of dying, depriving them of their expected lustful enjoyment: "Those who had been concerned in the joke were now sorry they had pushed it so far; however, the anxiety [...] was relieved by his returning to himself" (De Cervantes, 1605/1615, p. 710).

Often, an experience of imminent death produces total dependence on one's savior. Whether we call it Stockholm syndrome or identification with the aggressor, this addictive link will take time to loosen, because it is related to the wellspring of life in newborns. Unless another being can be counted on to wait for you, outside the hell of brutes. Sancho's steadfast donkey is all he needs to help him recover the boundaries of time: "He asked what o'clock it was [...]. He said no more, and in silence began to dress himself, while all watched him, waiting to see what the haste with which he was putting on his clothes meant." Without uttering a word, Sancho "proceeded to the stable, [...] and going up to Dapple [...] gave him a loving kiss on the forehead" (De Cervantes, 1605/1615, p. 712). It was out of the question to spend any more energy on behalf of his prosecutors.

In the face of their ferocity, the ass is the only reliable other for the survival of Sancho's psyche. A motor of transference, intended from the beginning, along with Rocinante, to carry the Quixotic dynamic, he is now promoted to the position of *therapon*, in the absence of Don Quixote. Dapple has now reached the pinnacle of achievement. Thanks to him, Sancho's bolstered spirits express themselves in a long sentence worthy of Proust:

> Come along, comrade and friend and partner of my toils and sorrows; when I was with you and had no cares to trouble me except mending your harness and feeding your little carcass, [...] but since I left you, and mounted the towers of ambition and pride,

> a thousand miseries, a thousand troubles and four thousand anxieties have entered into my soul.
>
> (De Cervantes, 1605/1615, p. 721)

Like Cervantes, the old warrior and slave, Sancho must purify his soul of the agony of living death. He fixes the packsaddle on the ass, mounts him, and rides off: "Make way, gentlemen, and let me go back to my old freedom; let me go look for my past life, and captain myself up from this present death" (De Cervantes, 1605/1615, p. 721).

Proust testifies to the same experience, after a brush with death. At the end of *Time Regained*, he describes how the idea of "a form which normally, is invisible, the form of Time" came to him once "the idea or death installed itself permanently in [him]" (Proust, 1927). "And often I asked myself not only whether there was still time but whether I was in a condition to accomplish my work. Illness which had rendered me a service by making me die to the world [...] was now perhaps going to save me from idleness" (Proust, 1927).

The quasi-mystical tone of the author of *In Search of Lost Time*, not long before his actual death, evokes the message Cervantes asked us to pass on to the forger. Whatever the distortions inflicted upon the work, Proust says, his ultimate Dulcinea remains a source of renewal and joy:

> I say that the cruel law of art is that beings die and that we ourselves must die after we have exhausted suffering so that the grass, not of oblivion but of eternal life, should grow, fertilised by works upon which generations to come will gaily picnic without care of those who sleep beneath it.

But first, Proust renounced the world, and Sancho will as well.

No!

This renouncement, after all the suffering endured, will involve for Sancho the passage through a purgatory space worthy of the rituals of ancient mysteries. The Latin author Apuleius depicts those of the second century AD, through the adventures of *The Golden Ass*, in which the donkey plays an essential role.

As he is about to leave, Sancho makes a speech that does not seem very revolutionary, and reiterates the motto of the Brotherhood of Wine-Growers—sung during their festival, four times in a century—in the Vevey region, on the banks of the Geneva Lake: "To each his craft, to each his specialty". Sancho comes to the same conclusion: "each of us is best following the trade he was born to". He claims none of the benefits acquired during his government: "naked I was born, naked I find myself, I neither lose nor gain". What counts is his action: "Stand aside, and let me go" (De Cervantes, 1605/1615, p. 722).

Regal and solitary, "he says what he does and does what he says", like Horton, Dr Seuss' elephant. Sustained only by his ancestry and descendants, he proclaims: "I am of the breed of the Panzas, and they are every one of them obstinate, and if they once say 'odds', odds it must be, no matter if it is evens, in spite of all the world."

Refusal to consent to voluntary servitude is summed up in two letters: No! Cervantes already told us when the convicts were set free. Jean Cassou, his French translator after the Second World War, insists on this point in *La Mémoire courte* (Short Memory): "But what is this Resistance if not, each time, the first stammerings of the conscience which refuses to consent to the obvious and fights for the improbable, even the impossible" (Cassou, 1953, p. 47).

Despite the slogans of future ducal courts that will attempt to lay claim to the Cervantian "no", Sancho's "no" is rooted in loyalty to his crazy master, "in whose society he was happier than in being governor of all the islands in the world" (De Cervantes, 1605/1615, p. 711).

"Half glad, half sad", Sancho disdains the approval of the henchmen who try to hold him back so that he may render an account of his mission. Determined not to answer to anyone but the duke, who appointed him, he embraced them before departing without complaint, leaving them "filled with admiration not only at his remarks, but at his firm and sensible resolution".

The only thing he requests is some barley for Dapple and half a loaf of bread and some cheese for himself. Nothing else matters. In his Discourse, also called the *Against-One,* La Boétie does not beat about the bush either, and tells the people that all they have to do is refuse to serve and take a side step to escape the grip of the tyrant: "I do not ask that you place hands upon the tyrant to topple him over, but simply that you support him no longer, then you will behold him, like a great Colossus whose pedestal has been pulled away, fall of his own weight and break in pieces" (La Boétie, 1548).

Far from trying to take the place of power, Sancho is content to leave. He says "no", "in spite of all the world", in order to be free to practise his profession of *therapon*, "the trade he was born to". He has refused the obvious and turned towards the improbable and the impossible.

Towards rebuilding the plural body

The duke and duchess were appalled that they had not been informed of Sancho's departure, and outraged to see how little he cared about their reaction. Because they are nothing without the media, the governor's resignation stuns them. Not only did this news go unreported, but it was not picked up by their spy network.

Indeed, Sancho did not bother to find out "whether it was island, city, town, or village that he governed he never troubled himself to inquire". His master had warned him never to look for the motives of perverse enchanters, but rather get away from them! Still, his troubles are not over. Having extricated himself from the ducal schemes, he runs into them again in the wider field of his country.

History enters the novel, by way of a meeting with six German pilgrims, who are in fact smugglers crossing the Pyrenees. One of them is his neighbour Ricote, the Arab shopkeeper of his village, banished from Spain by the edicts signed by King Philip III to expel the Moriscos, between 1609 and 1614. As a consequence, Spain was deprived of its active population of merchants and craftsmen. The provinces of Aragon, where the action takes place, lost a third of their population, which had been authorised to stay in Spain in 1492 after the Reconquista, provided they converted to Catholicism and spoke Spanish. Cervantes mentions several times that Ricote speaks perfect Castilian.

A picnic is quickly organised: bread, salt, cheese, olives, and caviar from the East, "a great thirst-wakener"; fortunately, there was no lack of wine, and they all "captained their arms and *botas* aloft, the mouths placed in their mouths, and all eyes fixed on heaven just as if they were taking aim at it" (De Cervantes, 1605/1615, p. 716). Once they were sated, Ricote told Sancho about his people's "terror and dismay" (De Cervantes, 1605/1615, p. 716) when the edict was suddenly issued against them, adding that at first he had trouble believing it would be enforced.

Today's illegal immigrants find themselves in the same situation. Ricote left Spain alone, intending to find a place where his family could come later; he finally settled in Augsburg, where the inhabitants enjoyed "liberty of conscience" (De Cervantes, 1605/1615, p. 717). Cervantes' condemnation of the forced separation of families expelled to Algeria, where they were unwanted, is unequivocal. Ricote describes the smuggling which, under the guise of pilgrimage, served to take money out of Spain. Ricote "cannot understand [...] why my wife and daughter should have gone to Barbary rather than to France" (De Cervantes, 1605/1615, p. 718). Sancho gave him the explanation he needs. Government employees at the border stole all their valuables, without further ado.

The facts are related without comment. Yet Sancho refuses to help his neighbour dig up the treasure he buried in his garden, despite the promise of a bribe. Traumatised by the recent violence which, as he says, makes one lose "rest and sleep, and even one's food", he narrates the departure of Ricote's wife and daughter; a scene which "made me weep myself, though I am not much given to tears commonly" (De Cervantes, 1605/1615, p. 719). His neighbour learns, incidentally, that his daughter has fallen in love with a rich young Castilian, but remains unconcerned, because "the Morisco women seldom or never engage in amours with the old Christians".

Time was to prove him wrong. This story, soon to be buried with Sancho in the bowels of the Earth, would re-emerge in Barcelona in a reviviscence of the piracy on the Mediterranean Sea, which led Miguel de Cervantes and his brother Rodrigo into slavery.

Lessons of darkness

"No man ever steps in the same river twice", says the pre-Socratic philosopher quoted by Cide Hamete.

After leaving his old neighbour, and still hoping to resume his previous life, Sancho falls into another trap. It is night. As he is looking for a place to sleep, he feels the earth opening up under his feet, and "he and Dapple [stumble] into a deep dark hole that [lies] among some very old buildings". It is, in a way, his own cave of Montesinos, but much more sinister, where his ass lands with his master sitting on him, fortunately "without [...] any hurt or damage whatever" (De Cervantes, 1605/1615, p. 720).

Cervantes does not deny the bitterness of freedom, when escape leaves the one who got away with a feeling of emptiness. No longer resisting the ruthless other bent on destroying him, he now has nothing to cling to. His dreams burst like soap bubbles. Still, Sancho's first concern is for his dear companion's safety, for "he heard how pathetically and dolefully [he] was bemoaning himself, [...] for in truth he was not in a very good case".

The unforgettable memory of his recent agony increases Sancho's solitude, as if, once out of hell, purgatory is no less distressful. He imagines a pit full of monstrous chthonic deities, "toads and addlers" (De Cervantes, 1605/1615, p. 721), no less disgusting than the creatures swimming in the Lake of Boiling Pitch. Buried alive, with no one to hear him, he is threatened with slow death again: "Here must we perish with hunger, my ass and myself, if indeed we don't die first, he of his bruises and injuries, and I of grief and sorrow."

He even anticipates some future time when archaeologists will dig up "[his] bones [...], picked clean, white and polished, and [his] good Dapple's with them", like in the tomb of a Celtic chief, buried with his mount. The plural body of their intermingled bones will then resurface to testify to their loyalty for all eternity. Like the bones of the *Grimsby Chums*—twenty English soldiers from the small port of Grimsby discovered recently near Arras, buried with their arms interlocked during the 1917 offensive, at the front line (Desfossés, 2009): "by that, perhaps, it will be found out who we are, at least by such as have heard that Sancho Panza never separated from his ass, nor his ass from Sancho Panza" (De Cervantes, 1605/1615, p. 728).

Delivered in the future perfect tense, the funeral eulogy praises an ancient deity celebrated in the Middle Ages between Christmas and New Year's Eve. During that week, the "Feast of the Ass" coincided with the "Feast of the Fools" and the "Feast of the Children" commemorating the Massacre of the Innocents. In the same week, which had been previously dedicated to the Roman Saturnales—when slaves, often called children, took power—women in Savoy were officially allowed to rule the household.

As wise as the learned Master Aliboron, the donkey is also endowed with the infallible memory of the hero of children's books—Monsieur Cadichon (Countess de Ségur, 2011) and Culotte the Donkey (Bosco, 1978)—because his great ears allow him to hear the invisible. In the poem "The Toad", Victor Hugo celebrates the donkey who spares a toad stuck in the mud of the road, after it has been tormented by a group of children, the young Victor among them (Hugo, 1859). No longer part of our landscapes, real donkeys have left a great void in the lives of modern children mesmerised by screens.

"I love the gentle donkey ..."

"J'aime l'âne si doux, marchant le long des houx" (... walking beside the hollies) is a famous verse by the French poet Francis Jammes (1898). In the Later Roman Empire, the "golden ass" awakened the erotic passions of a Roman matron. More recently, another donkey aroused such tenderness in the heart of his mistress that she immortalised him in a nursery rhyme that has soothed many sorrows: "Mon âne, mon âne, a bien mal à la tête":

> My donkey, my donkey, his head aches so upon it
> The doctor has told him to wear a woolen bonnet,
> [...] And eat a lot of lollipops.

In a 1517 poem, Machiavelli himself changes into a donkey, so he can enjoy kicking and farting to his heart's content (Ordine, 1996). But the role in which the donkey excels is that of messenger of infernal deities. Hermaneus, from the name of the god Hermes, means "ass driver". His intrusive eloquence inspired Cervantes to imagine the braying contest. But now, he is Sancho's *therapon*, in the larger sense of the word, which means not only "the second in combat" but also, "the ritual double", in charge of funeral duties. Here, at the approach of death, his braying will, on the contrary, save both their lives.

In this poetic role, the donkey's impressive phallic and vocal organs embody the return from death to life. He has, like Orpheus, shamanic powers. Thanks to him, the young man changed into a donkey in Apuleius' *Golden Ass*—also called *The Metamorphoses*—crosses the dark underside of society and understands everything he hears, without saying anything.

Lamenting their fate, Sancho promises Dapple to crown him with a laurel wreath that will make him a poet laureate: "and his ass listened to him, but answered him never a word".

The situation is critical. When day dawns, it becomes clear that it will be impossible to get out of the pit, and the panic reaches its peak: "I cannot bear being buried alive any longer, and I'm dying of fear."

Confronting death regenerates his psyche, which abandons the carcass of his old ego with its "follies and fancies", and advances, lighter, towards life, albeit at a slow pace, for Dapple "was scarcely able to keep [his feet]". The ass eats the piece of bread shared according to the survival rules of the plural body in war time, which demand that the other be nourished first, before thinking of oneself: "he gave it to the ass, to whom it was not unwelcome, saying to him as if he understood him, 'With bread all sorrows are less'" (De Cervantes, 1605/1615, p. 721).

The sacrificial pit is transformed once again into a cave for speleologists. Sancho sees the light at the end of a tunnel, into which he crawls on all fours, reversing their roles and widening the opening, so that his donkey, pulled by the halter, could pass through it. While they advance, the Lake of Boiling Pitch comes to his mind, where Don Quixote "[came] out of this darkness and imprisonment into some blooming meadow" (De Cervantes, 1605/1615, p. 721). More pessimistic, Sancho expects the earth to open up under his feet at any moment, and when he finally "perceived a dim light", he believed he was on the road to the other world.

But, by the merest chance—for "the compliance of chance is irrefutable" (McGuire,1974), as Freud says in a 1909 letter to Jung, and undeniable in case of a catastrophe—Don Quixote's path crosses the underground path of his buried squire on that particular morning.

Hee-haw

"It came to pass, then, that having sallied forth one morning to practise and exercise himself"—for next day's duel to save the duena's honour—"as he was putting Rocinante through his paces or pressing him to the charge, he brought his feet so close to a pit that but for reining him in tightly it would have been impossible for him to avoid falling into it".

The horse's magic hooves draw forth cries from the bowels of the earth. Don Quixote, above, recognises the resounding voice of the donkey and exclaims: "Famous testimony! [...] I know that bray as well as if I was its mother" (De Cervantes, 1605/1615, p. 723).

A fine tribute to the role of the donkey as a transporter of souls from this word to the beyond, and in the other direction. Then the knight hears Sancho's voice, which he first believes to be that of his ghost. "it suggested itself to his mind that Sancho must be dead, and that his soul was in torment down there". As an analyst familiar with the traumatic spheres of death, Don Quixote speaks to the one who fell through the cracks of time, very reasonably offering, "as [his] profession is to give aid and succor to those that need it in this world", to place himself in his service, since his role "will also extend to aiding and succoring the distressed of the other [world], who cannot help themselves" (De Cervantes, 1605/1615, p. 722).

Don Quixote, *the therapon*, also remembers, like the donkey, his ritual role that includes funeral duties. He starts by checking the identity of the soul in torment: "tell me who thou art, [...] because, if thou art my squire Sancho Panza, and art dead, since the devils have not carried thee off ...".

The invention of Purgatory in the twelfth century (Le Goff, 1986)—where a door finally opens between the living and the dead—makes it possible to communicate with the deceased, like pagans did in their ceremonies, without incurring the wrath of the Church. Sancho protests in vain that he is no ghost, since he "[has] never died in all [his] life"; the only reliable proof of life is the braying of the donkey, who cannot lie about his origins.

The primary opposition, hee/haw, has the same value for Don Quixote as the *fort/da* (gone/there) of Freud's grandson has for Freud (1920). It serves to tame absence and death. This primordial braying, recognised at once by the knight, makes sense of Sancho's disappearance and brings him out of the black hole into which he had vanished without a trace. By contrast, the duke and duchess—urged by Don Quixote to send rescuers equipped with ropes and tackle—could not understand what had happened. Even if they had heard the hee-haw of the donkey, it would not have meant much to them since, being primarily interested in themselves, they are more dumb than the animal: "they could easily understand his having fallen, from the confirmatory circumstances of the cave which had been in existence there from time immemorial; but they could not imagine how he had quit the government without their receiving any intimation of his coming" (De Cervantes, 1605/1615, p. 723).

If we follow the text closely, we can see that Cervantes is referring to the traditional route of ancient ceremonial practices, a path that required time to travel across, to give words a chance to regain their weight. Don Quixote greets Sancho upon his return from his "vision quest", and authenticates his journey with an irrefutable argument: "keep a safe conscience and let them say what they like, for trying to stop slanderers' tongues is like trying to put gates to open plain" (De Cervantes, 1605/1615, p. 724).

The slanderers cannot prevent the former governor from giving an account of his government to the duke and the duchess, in the form of his favourite refrain: "I entered naked, and naked I find myself; I neither lose nor gain. […] yesterday morning I left the island as I found it […], I asked no loan of anybody, nor did I try to fill my pocket."

But this time, his condemnation of corruption includes a resounding refusal. It echoes the "no" of the young La Boétie, through which he gained Montaigne's friendship: "Obviously there is no need of fighting to overcome this single tyrant, for he is automatically defeated if the country refuses consent to its own enslavement" (La Boétie, 1548). Here, Sancho the jester expresses the refusal to consent through a leaping gesture:

> kissing your worships' feet, and imitating the game of the boys when they say, "leap thou, and give me one", I take a leap out of the government and pass into the service of my master Don Quixote, for after all, though in it I eat my bread in fear and trembling, at any rate I take my fill; and for my part, so long as I'm full, it's all alike to me whether it's with carrots or with partridges.
>
> (De Cervantes, 1605/1615, p. 724)

Kafka was going to use the same image to speak of his writing. In his view, "To write is to jump outside the line of the assassins" (1925).

Jumping into the fray

Don Quixote, Rocinante, Sancho, and Dapple are reunited at last, in preparation of a duel worthy of *The Three Musketeers*—one for all and all for one! A multitude of people flocked to see the encounter, a rare event, since "the decree of the holy Council […] prohibited all challenges of the sort". After the austerity of the underground cave, the decorum of the tournaments, which had killed a king of France in the previous century, is very alluring. In the fray, Don Quixote's opponent, unbeknownst to him, will be a lackey, because the true felon has fled to Flanders for fear of having Dona Rodriguez for a mother-in-law.

Drum-rolls and trumpet-calls resound, the ground shakes under horses' hooves, "the hearts of the gazing crowd were full of anxiety".

Don Quixote set out "at the highest speed Rocinante was capable of", to meet his enemy, who "never stirred a step from the spot where he was posted" (De Cervantes, 1605/1615, p. 728). Stupefaction! Love at first sight. Tosilos, the lackey is fascinated by the duena's daughter. Long before Victor Hugo's Ruy Blas, Tosilos is "the earthworm in love with a star". Indeed, Eros, ready to play his trump card to save Psyche from Venus' wrath once again, has shot a well-aimed arrow which nailed to the spot the love-crazed lackey. Deaf to the furore of the duel, the young man foils the ducal plot by speaking directly to the duena: "Senora, I am willing to marry your daughter, and I have no wish to obtain by strife and fighting what I can obtain in peace and without any risk to my life" (De Cervantes, 1605/1615, p. 728).

Don Quixote takes back his word at once: "As that is the case I am released and absolved from my promise; let them marry by all means": "amazed and extremely angry", the duke is about to have a fit. Unexpectedly, Tosilos and the duena have leaped "outside the line of the assassins". Of course, the plaintiffs made a great outcry when they saw the face of the lackey, but the sincere passion of youth triumphed over false excitement.

Don Quixote resolves the incident by invoking, as usual, "those wicked enchanters who persecute me" and who changed the identity of the seducer. For once, all is well that ends well, and the would-be bride agrees: "I had rather be the lawful wife of a lackey than the cheated mistress of a gentleman; though he who played me false is nothing of the kind" (De Cervantes, 1605/1615, p. 729).

And Cervantes takes this opportunity to make a heartfelt remark on crowd psychology, inferred from the reaction of the spectators:

> the greater number were vexed and disappointed at finding that the combatants they had been so anxiously waiting for had not battered one another to pieces, just as they boys are disappointed when the man they are waiting to see hanged does not come out, because the prosecution or the court has pardoned him.
>
> (De Cervantes, 1605/1615, p. 729)

Today, "the greater number" goes home just as disappointed, but can happily watch television shows just as sad and cruel as the show they missed. Of course, the Quixotic action does not prevent Tosilos' fairy tale from going sour. The young lackey will return—like Andrés, the shepherd in the first novel, who later cursed the knight for having saved him (De Cervantes, 1605/1615, p. 574). When Tosilos meets Don Quixote by chance eighty pages further (De Cervantes, 1605/1615, p. 789), he informs the knight of the retaliation inflicted on him and on the two women. Cervantes underscores the point by saying that expecting perverts to relinquish their aims is "to ask pears from the elm tree".

But no matter! As long as at some point particular subjects triumph over those who treat them like objects, the trace of this moment will be registered by someone and have a chance of being transmitted. Who knows, perhaps the duena's daughter who was sent to a convent will meet an intelligent Teresa d'Avila or her friend Luisa, the sister of Cervantes, prioress of the Carmelite convent in Alcala. In any case, the political scope of Quixotic action goes beyond social status. Hannah Arendt points out that the two spheres, social and political, must not be confused. Don Quixote clearly asserts it as well: "[he] now felt it right to quit a life of such idleness as he was leading in the castle, for he fancied that he was making himself sorely missed by suffering himself to remain shut up and inactive amid the countless luxuries and enjoyments his hosts lavished upon him" (De Cervantes, 1605/1615, p. 730).

He too jumps out of the servitude of a "generous" hospitality that has driven him to forget his profession. The memory of his former freedom urges him to find his own centre again. He belongs to "the few" described by La Boétie, who "like Ulysses on land and sea constantly seeking the smoke of his chimney, cannot prevent themselves from peering about for their natural privileges and from remembering their ancestors and their former ways" (La Boétie, 1548).

*Song of departure**

Don Quixote was leaving a life of idleness for which "he would have to render a strict account to heaven", as Ulysses did when he tore himself away from the charms of Circe (Homer, 8th century BC, chant X). As early as 1582, Giordano Bruno, the "academic from no academy", wandered through Europe like a Don Quixote. In his *Cantus Circaeus*, he announced the crisis of a world struggling with "vulgar and inconsistent things, although seductive in appearance" (Levergeois, 1995).

**Le Chant du Départ*, title of a French Revolutionary song.

Bruno's works, like those of Cervantes, are visionary. A forerunner of Aby Warburg who declared "God is in the details", Bruno's poem *De triplici minimo*, written in 1591 in Paris, asserts that "divine nature is manifest in trinkets". Moreover, Bruno prefigured psychoanalysis when he invented an art of memory, *De umbris idearum*, in order to "find traces of the real, thanks to the tool of association of verbal memory, which can make meaningful links between syllables and images".

Indeed, Don Quixote has not forgotten what he owes, not to dukes, who took more than their share, but to his profession of arms and letters, as well as to his father's stain, Cervantes' *mancha*. His madness is a memory that does not forget, which impelled him to undertake his adventures, rather than languish at home or luxuriate in the castle (he is about to leave). He felt he owed a strict accounting to heaven, "and so [...] he asked the duke and duchess to grant him permission to take his departure" (De Cervantes, 1605/1615, p. 729).

But just when he and Sancho are on the threshold of freedom, the stain is brought back when rumours accuse both of them of theft. Cervantes, who remembers only too well—from his experiences in Algiers and later in Spain—the suspicions that arise in hostage negotiations, does not nurture any illusions about the media coverage of their liberation.

The day they leave their luxurious hostel, which Sancho will always miss, despite his protestations of moral purity, a comical song sung by Altisidora attempts to discredit them. Before all those who "were watching [them] from the corridors", she accuses them of having stolen three kerchiefs and a pair of garters (De Cervantes, 1605/1615, p. 731). Taken by surprise, the duchess treats Don Quixote like a rogue, a vulgar picaro suspected of fetishism—given the garter—and uses terms evocative of a brothel. The duke goes even further, saying: "Restore her garters, or else I defy you to mortal combat" (De Cervantes, 1605/1615, p. 732).

Sex and blood are commonly used as political trump cards with entertainment value, when the media have nothing else to say. Don Quixote is sick of it: "God forbid, that I should draw my sword against your illustrious person from which I have received such great favors." Sancho will give back the kerchiefs he admits he stole. The master defends his squire:

> as to the garters that is impossible, for I have not got them, neither has he; and if your handmaiden here will look in her hiding places, depend upon it she will find them. I have never been a thief, my

> lord duke, nor do I mean to be so long as I live, if God cease not to have me in his keeping.
>
> (De Cervantes, 1605/1615, pp. 732–733)

Despite the public disgrace, they do not try to justify themselves. The simple gesture of farewell has political scope of another nature, linked with symbolic debt—a notion unknown at the castle. Thus, Don Quixote speaks of his profession as something for which accounting must be rendered, and of his idleness as intolerable waste. He knows that he owes his power of regeneration to his father. By contrast, the ducal power keeps those indebted to it through corruption in a total state of dependency.

These two forms of exchange have nothing in common. Don Quixote shows the crowd gathered to see the two heroes leave how to free oneself from a perverted social link.

CHAPTER FIVE

On the road again!

Giordano Bruno's error

Giordano Bruno did not have the good fortune of getting away from the castle of perversion. After a European odyssey, *andante!*, that lasted nearly fifteen years—between 1578 and 1592—he returned to Venice at the invitation of a progressive patrician, Giovanni Mocenigo (Lavergeois, 1995, p. 474) who handed him over to the Holy Office. Condemned to be burned at the stake in Rome, with all his writings, he mounted the gibbet erected in the middle of Campo de' Fiori in 1600, after eight years of imprisonment.

Born in 1548, he was one year younger than Cervantes. As he declared before his judges, he was the son of a soldier. His father was a standard-bearer in Naples, in the army Miguel joined when he arrived in Italy in 1566.

That year, Naples was devastated by an earthquake followed by floods and famine. Giordano Bruno had been in the city for a year, in a Dominican monastery from which he fled in 1576, because he had disobeyed the ban on reading Erasmus. Rabelais had escaped earlier, for the same reason, from his Franciscan monastery.

When, in 1575, Cervantes was captured by Barbary pirates, and taken to Algiers as a slave, Giordano Bruno was setting out on his long journey. He passed through Genoa where the plague raged, killing Titian, and in 1578 was excommunicated in Geneva by the Calvinists. After spending some time in Toulouse, in 1581 he went on to Paris, where he stayed five years at the Court of Henri III, the last monarch of the Valois dynasty, who appointed him lecturer extraordinaire at the Royal College. There, he wrote his famous play *The Candle-Bearer*, which features capeadors: the cape thieves supposed to be at the origin of the Neapolitan Camorra (Saviano, 2008).

In 1586, after a quarrel, he was forced to leave Paris and went to Wittemberg, Luther's home town; from there, he went to the Court of Rudolph II in Prague, and afterwards to Tübingen. In 1590, he was excommunicated once again in Helmstedt, this time by the Lutherans. In 1591, for the Frankfurt Book Fair, he published the texts *De Minimo* and *De Immenso*, written while he was in Paris, in Quixotic style:

> But we, at the mercy of contradictory events, and although we have fought the vagaries of fortune since our youth, have kept undiminished the resolve and boldness which give us strength and, as God is our witness, we have never idled or tarried, but have always defended against the signs of evil by despising them; accordingly, nothing can cause us to fear death, and we have never surrendered the power of our mind to any mortal.
>
> (Lavergeois, 1995, p. 456)

Giordano Bruno (1950) praised the donkey as well, speaking of "positive assness" characterised by perseverance, which he contrasts with "negative assness", being pedantic and arrogant. That same year, 1591—a year before Cervantes was imprisoned in Seville—his farewell address to his Wittemberg hosts resonates with familiar tones. He thanks them for defending the freedom of philosophical thought, brought to their city by "a person of no name, fame or value among you, supported by no prince's praise, distinguished by no outward trappings such as the vulgar are wont to admire, a fugitive from the Gallic tumults".

The events surrounding his fatal error of returning to Venice at the request of the traitor bring to mind the two Cervantean heroes who will be brought back to the castle *manu militari*, at the end of the novel, to be delivered to a make-believe Inquisition. For Giordano Bruno, the sinister enactment is all too real. Before being burned at the stake on 17 February 1600, he told his executioners: "Perchance you who pronounce my sentence are in greater fear than I who receive it" (Ordine, 1996).

His death sent shockwaves throughout Europe, and must have made a strong impression on Cervantes, as it did on young Descartes, who put off publishing his treaty *The Meteors* for fear of suffering the same fate.

"Ciao! Ciao! Ciao!"

Don Quixote and Sancho have left the castle on their respective mounts, without looking back, and feeling light: "When Don Quixote saw himself in open country, free, and relieved from the attentions of Altisidora, he felt at his ease, and in fresh spirits" (De Cervantes, 1605/1615, p. 734).

Turning to Sancho, he says:

> Freedom, Sancho, is one of the most precious gifts that heaven has bestowed upon men; no treasures that the earth holds buried or the sea conceals can compare with it; for freedom, as for honor, life may and should be ventured; and on the other hand, captivity is the greatest evil that can fall to the lot of man.
>
> (De Cervantes, 1605/1615, p. 734)

He knows what he is talking about, since he has become the forger's spoils, just as his father had been a treasure delivered by the sea to pirates, and then risked his life four times to escape. Although much more comfortable, the ducal castle made them no less captive than the ransom slaves held by Hassan Pacha, the powerful dey of Algiers:

> I say this, Sancho, because thou hast seen the good cheer, the abundance we have enjoyed in this castle we are leaving; well then, amid those dainty banquets and snow-cooled beverages I felt as though I were undergoing the straits of hunger, because I did not enjoy them with the same freedom as if they had been mine own.
>
> (De Cervantes, 1605/1615, p. 734)

Don Quixote can finally analyse his unspeakable anguish while he is enjoying all the comforts of the castle. It comes from the theft of their story, from their portrayal as living the high life, showing off and having fun.

This situation also creates a debt, as illustrated in *The Godfather* (Coppola, 1972):

> the sense of being under an obligation to return benefits and favors received is a restraint that checks the independence of the spirit. Happy he, to whom heaven has given a piece of bread for which he is not bound to give thanks to any but heaven itself!

There follows a quotation from the Beatitudes Sermon, describing the lilies of the field, the birds, and all the creatures whose bounty is given by heaven. But Sancho has not left the castle empty-handed. The majordomo has given the squire, unbeknownst to Don Quixote, "two hundred gold crowns [...] in a little purse which [Sancho carries] next to [his] heart, like a warming plaster or comforter" (De Cervantes, 1605/1615, p. 734).

With good reason, for he doubts that they will ever find a palace like this again, but most likely only "roadside inns where they'll cudgel us". No matter! The free flow of their talking cure, interrupted some two hundred pages back, is taken up again as if nothing had happened. Paying no heed to the threat hanging over the knight—Carrasco is about to form an alliance with the dukes—they set out on the road again, *andante*.

A happy omen

Their first steps on the road of freedom lead them to an encounter with sculpted images, gilded with gold leaf and carried under sheets. For once, a happy omen! They were figures of saints, who had been famous knights, each one mounted on his Rocinante: Saint Paul, Saint Martin, Saint George, and Saint James. Treasures from the deepest reaches of Spain, they travelled on the roads, like the itinerant artists who created them, as described later, in the eighteenth-century diary of a sculptor from the Piedmont mountains (Giraldi, 1998), who walked from village to village on both sides of the Alps, to sculpt and regild the altarpieces of baroque churches in Savoy.

"Let the money they cost speak for [their quality]", says the peasant Don Quixote asked about them, curious to see the sculptures under the sheets.

> getting up from his dinner he went and uncovered the first image, which proved to be one of Saint George on horseback with a serpent writhing at his feet and the lance thrust down its throat [...]. The whole group was one blaze of gold, as the saying is.
>
> (De Cervantes, 1605/1615, p. 735)

By contrast, the self-appointed stars at the castle seem dull, compared to these mythical companions. In ancient mysteries, the unveiling of deities revitalised depleted souls. *All my relatives!* say the Sioux people during their ceremonies. The knight recognises fellow knights-errant in the sculpted images. Does this mean that he too has defeated the dragon? We shall soon have the answer, given beforehand by Giordano Bruno and some others, for whom the true target of the lance is the one who wields it.

Before venturing into such mystical territories, Sancho thanks providence for "one of the sweetest and pleasantest" adventures they have ever had. It is a genuine *kledôn*: a fortunate accident unrelated to common reason.

The discussion naturally turns to how best to profit from such a lucky circumstance without falling into foolish credulity. Altisidora and her pranks have now been left far behind, but the pleasure of her acquaintance remains on their minds. Sancho still doesn't understand how she could have had a crush on his master. No matter how often he looked at him "from the sole of [his] foot to the topmost hair of [his] head, [he saw] more to frighten one than to make one fall in love" (De Cervantes, 1605/1615, p. 737).

Don Quixote agrees: "I [...] perceive clearly enough that I am not beautiful."

His appearance is, in fact, as we say in French, "a remedy against love". But he claims to possess a certain beauty of soul. In the myth of Apuleius, Psyche's beauty made Venus insanely envious. For it sprung from what she did not know about herself, from the unconscious to which divinities have no access, as the knight astutely remarks:

> I take it as a happy omen, brothers, to have seen what I have; for these saints and knights were of the same profession as myself, which is the calling of arms; only there is this difference between them and me, that they were saints, and fought with divine weapons, and I

> am a sinner and fight with human ones. They won heaven by force of arms [...]; and I, so far, know not what I have won by dint of my suffering.
>
> (De Cervantes, 1605/1615, pp. 735–736)

Fortified by all these knights he regards as his patron saints, Don Quixote will revisit, like in transgenerational analysis, other traumas of Cervantes' life, in order to inscribe them and then break away.

Back to the pastoral romance

> While engaged in this discourse they were making their way through a wood that lay beyond the road, when suddenly, without expecting anything of the kind, Don Quixote found himself caught in some nets of green cord stretched from one tree to another [...] just as he was about to press forward and break through all, suddenly from among some trees two shepherdesses of surpassing beauty presented themselves to his sight—or at least damsels dressed like shepherdesses, save that their jerkins and sayas were of fine brocade.
>
> (De Cervantes, 1605/1615, p. 738)

A far cry from Teresa Panza's grey smock.

Here they are again, caught in a pastoral web. These beautiful blonde maidens, whose "years to all appearances were not under fifteen nor above eighteen", seem to have stepped right out of the *Galatea*. Thirty years have passed since Cervantes published his first six books in 1582. Others had been promised, but nothing materialised, especially after Cervantes landed in a Seville prison in 1592. To see shepherdesses take hostage the hero who has left them behind was in line with the family history.

Don Quixote had always been ambivalent about the characters of pastoral romances. He had been charmed by the shepherdess Marcela and the goatherd Pedro, but he had fought with another goatherd enamoured of his goat (De Cervantes, 1605/1615, Vol. I, chapters XII, XIII, LI, LII), and was now enchanted once again. Sancho was "filled with amazement" and Don Quixote was "fascinated" by so much beauty: "[The] spectacle [...] made the sun halt in his course to behold them, and held all four in a strange silence."

In case we are not familiar with the universe of pastoral romance, one of the shepherdesses breaks the silence to provide two indispensable references to the ignorant reader: the famous Spanish poet Garcilaso de las Vegas and "the most excellent Camoens" of Portugal, a major source of inspiration for Cervantes' Galatea, who was about to marry a Portuguese shepherd when her author dropped her. Don Quixote returns to the pastoral style again: "Of a truth, fairest lady, Actaeon when he beheld Diana bathing in a stream could not have been more [...] wonderstruck [...]; and if, instead of taking up, as they probably do, but a small space, these nets took up the whole surface of the globe, I would seek out new worlds through which to pass, so as not to break them" (De Cervantes, 1605/1615, p. 739). Thereupon, he introduces himself and is greeted with great enthusiasm.

In the midst of the feverish literary reunion of the brother, Don Quixote, with his older sister Galatea, the most passionate phrases are pronounced by one of the shepherdesses: "Ah! Friend of my soul, what great good fortune has befallen us! Seest thou this gentleman we have before us?" There follows a string of superlatives: "his is the most valiant and the most devoted and the most courteous gentleman in all the world". She has also read the history of his exploits.

The *locus amoenus* (pleasant place) described by Theocritus and Virgil has always been the ideal alternative to the corruption of civilisation. Peace and love! In France, the "Map of Tender"—an imaginary land—has just been situated in the Lignon River valley by the author of *L'Astrée* (1658), Honoré d'Urté, another soldier novelist who died in combat in 1625. In the following century, the nursery rhyme "Il pleut, il pleut, bergère, rentre tes blancs moutons" (The rains have come, shepherdess, bring in your white sheep) announced the roar of thunder at Versaille, in Queen Marie-Antoinette's hamlet. Later, in the nineteenth century, the desire for a return to nature led readers to Walden Pond, near Boston, where Thoreau had sought solitude in the woods, in a cabin belonging to Ralph Waldo Emerson. A century later, their great-grandchildren sparked the hippie movement in California, in part as a reaction to the Vietnam War and the traumas it inflicted.

Cervantes has no illusions about the political uses of pastoral decoys to trap the songs of nature in the greenery of ideology: "And now the gave was started, and the nets were filled with a variety of birds that deceived by the color fell into the danger they were flying from" (De Cervantes, 1605/1615, p. 739).

Cruelty is not absent from the pastoral romance. In fact, the *Galatea* starts with a crime and continues with the narration of a young man who became a hermit after being kidnapped by Barbary pirates on the Catalan shore. It speaks of rape and murder as well as a of desire, which "never attains its wishes", "for love and desire are different matters, for all we love we do not necessarily covet, or contrariwise" (De Cervantes, 1585, p. 194). In addition, Galatea discusses perversion, suicide, and even Oedipus: "Let none desire offspring, for Oedipus in blind rage killed his father" (De Cervantes, 1585, p. 194).

Indeed, aside from repressed desires, traumas are to be found everywhere. The attacks on ships by Ottoman pirates led by the Albanese renegade Arnaut Mami, who was to take Cervantes captive in 1575, are vividly described in *Galatea*: "This scene confounds the imagination when memory reverts to it" (De Cervantes, 1585, p. 235).

Exhausted, disillusioned, and traumatised, portraying himself as Lauso (De Cervantes, 1605/1615, p. 235), Cervantes chooses the pastoral genre in order to invent new signifiers to appease the Furies that haunt him since his return from war and slavery. As Jean Canavaggio points out, the aim of the pastoral novel is to *razonar cosas de amor* (give range to thoughts of love) (De Cervantes, 1605/1615, p. 819), and regain one's senses by finding the right word, since in both medieval and classical Spanish *razon* also means the "proper word".

Here, Cervantes comes up against the limits of classical psychoanalysis when it deals with trauma, when the symbolic chain suddenly breaks off. Other tools are needed to tame the Furies of traumatic revivals, to succeed in "taming wild thoughts", as Bion says (1997)—wild thoughts that stop the flow of time in its tracks.

Twenty years after the *Galatea*, Don Quixote was begotten to fight melancholia (Davoine, 2016), to proceed, with the surivivng images of his folly, beyond the point where the pastoral novel ended.

His fame arouses the admiration of the "elegant shepherds and shepherdesses" who are enacting eclogues depicting a life of innocence. Magnanimously, the knight offers to repay "the favor that has been extended to me" by praising them in Saragossa, where he is going. But he cannot stay long in the narrow confines of their make-believe universe. At that point, Sancho makes the blunder of "reasoning" about his madness: "Is it possible there is anyone in the world who will dare to say and swear that this master of mine is a madman?" (De Cervantes, 1605/1615, p. 740).

This discussion about labels and the "proper word" enrages Don Quixote, whose mission is not to argue about his diagnosis. Unexpectedly, he flies into a rage and takes us back to the good old times of his early adventures.

The myth of actaeon

We can bet that the knight sprung forth in the same manner, from Cervantes' toolbox, in the Seville prison where the latter was unable to write a sequel to *Galatea*, and was wondering if he was going mad. Don Quixote helped him to shake off his melancholia by reminding him, in the middle of total collapse, of the essential role of the Lady of his thoughts. He now delivers the same message to Sancho:

> Who asked thee to meddle in my affairs, or to inquire whether I am a wise man or a blockhead? [...] and in a great rage, and showing his anger plainly, [...] mounted on Rocinante [and] posted himself in the middle of a high road [to proclaim] that the beauty [...] enshrined in the nymphs that dwell in these meadows and groves surpass all upon earth, putting aside the lady of [his] heart, Dulcinea del Toboso.
>
> (De Cervantes, 1605/1615, pp. 740–741)

The reader understands now that Dulcinea has replaced Galatea. The knight's challenge, proclaimed "in the middle of [the] road" is not to argue about words, but to revive the source from which they arise, when the foundation of speech has been destroyed by brutes. And the brutes soon appear in person.

Just as he is making his public declaration, Don Quixote was knocked down by "fierce bulls", driven by true cowboys, gauchos, *vaqueros*, or herdsmen who hurled him to the ground when he refused to get out of the way. The whole procession "passed over Don Quixote and over Sancho, Rocinante and Dapple" (De Cervantes, 1605/1615, p. 741). A bullfighter from no bullring, facing a drove of bulls that overturned the "imitation Arcadia" and cancelled his speech, Don Quixote ran after the herd, "stumbling here and falling there".

When his *Don Quixote* was trampled underfoot by the *vulgum pecus* (vulgar herd), Cervantes too must have been tempted to run after the "rascally rabble". But now we have come to the crossroads where the tumultuous madness in the first novel has become exhausting and is no longer of use to the knight: "Weariness brought Don Quixote to a halt, and more enraged than avenged he sat down on the road to wait until Sancho, Rocinante and Dapple came up" (De Cervantes, 1605/1615, p. 742).

In fact, this pause marks the acquisition of a new wisdom, rediscovered in every era. Robert Musil discovered it in Paris, when he was violently trampled for his ideas. Having fled the Nazi regime, he had arrived in Paris from Vienna, to attend the congress focusing on the defence of culture against fascism, held at the Maison de la Mutualité in 1935. Because he dared—as Hannah Arendt would do fifteen years later—to equate the two totalitarian systems, he was shouted down by an enraged audience. He had ended his address by declaring in Quixotic manner: "Writers must defend their own integrity [...] without expecting any assistance from the State, which, whatever its political form, has recourse to culture only as a weapon that it uses to achieve its own mysterious ends" (Roditi, 1986).

Two years later, in Vienna, he gave a lecture entitled "On Stupidity", and then left Austria for Switzerland after the Anschluss. In 1942, the day he died of a heart attack in Geneva, he wrote, under the heading "Breaths of a Summer Day":

> "My heart was taken from out my breast", a mystic had said. [...] Time stood still, a thousand years weighed as lightly as the opening and closing of an eye ... [...] But if [...] you attain the highest selflessness, then finally outer and inner will touch each other as if a wedge that had split the world had popped out!
>
> (Musil, 1995, pp. 1327–1329)

Such a moment of awakening, which the knight will soon experience, was described by Eugen Herrigel as well, in his little book on the knightly art of archery in Japan:

> "Do you now understand", the Master asked me one day after a particularly good shot, "what I mean by: 'It shoots, It hits?'" "I'm afraid I don't understand anything any more at all," I answered, [...] "Is it I who draw the bow, or is it the bow that draws me [...]? Do I hit the goal, or does the goal hit me? [...] And even the need to separate has gone."
>
> (Herrigel, 1999)

Don Quixote, who aims for the target of healing his father's injured soul, becomes himself this target. And the arrow that hits him becomes Cervantes' pen and soul. On the last page of the novel, the pen speaks through a magnificent prosopopeia. The short interval separating the father and the son from their death shall henceforth be used to abolish the division separating the subject from the object standing between the author and his tale.

Death was Cervantes' companion, just as it was that of his favourite poets. The authors of pastoral romances, Camoëns and Montemajor, the author of *Diana*, were valiant warriors, as was Musil, who had been decorated during the First World War. To prepare the reader for this passage, the myth of Diana and Actaeon is invoked by Don Quixote during his encounter with the shepherdesses. In the myth, the hunter who glimpsed Diana bathing in the stream was changed into a deer and devoured by his own dogs. On that topic, Giordano Bruno's version of the myth asserts that in his frenzy, the hunter intent upon the capture of divine wisdom, recognises it in himself.

> Therefore, Actaeon, who with these thoughts searched for goodness, wisdom [...], once he was in their presence, ravished outside of himself by so much beauty, he became the prey of his own dogs and saw himself converted into the thing he was pursuing. Having already tracked down the divinity within himself, it was no longer necessary to hunt for it elsewhere.
>
> (Bruno, 1585)

In other words, "Become who you are!" But this principle of renunciation is not easy to accept. In fact, it pushes Don Quixote to the brink of suicide.

Anorexia

Although the two heroes resume their talking cure near "a clear limpid spring", Don Quixote is not really there: "Eat Sancho my friend, support life, which is of more consequence to thee than to me, and leave me to die under the pain of my thoughts and pressure of my misfortunes. I was born, Sancho, to live dying, and thou to die eating" (De Cervantes, 1605/1615, p. 743).

Unable to make him change his mind, "trampling every sort of good breeding under foot, [Sancho] began to stow away in his paunch the bread and cheese that came to his hand" (De Cervantes, 1605/1615, p. 743).

Clearly, the indifference of the rogues has disheartened Cervantes' son and his companion, as it had affected the father. Don Quixote confesses: "I looked forward to palms [...] and [...] I have this morning seen myself trampled on, kicked, and crushed by the feet of unclean and filthy animals" (De Cervantes, 1605/1615, p. 743).

So successful is the work of the forger and his friends that Don Quixote turns their malevolence against himself and becomes anorexic: "This thought blunts my teeth, paralyses my jaws, cramps my hands, and robs me of all appetite for food; so much so that I have a mind to let myself die of hunger, the cruelest death of all deaths" (De Cervantes, 1605/1615, p. 743).

The post-traumatic syndrome will come back ten chapters later, when they will pass through the same place again. Sancho refuses to give in to depression. His remedy is simple: food and sleep. "and you will see that when you awake you'll feel something better" (De Cervantes, 1605/1615, p. 743).

Tomorrow is another day, the saying goes, and indeed the next day they shall arrive at an inn a league off. In the meantime, Don Quixote attempts to pass his depression on to his *therapon* by asking him to whip himself to disenchant Dulcinea.

> Sancho, if thou wilt for me what I am going to tell thee my ease of mind would be more assured and my heaviness of heart not so great; and it is this; to go aside a little while I am sleeping in accordance with thy advice, and making bare thy carcass to the air, to give thyself three or four hundred lashes with Rocinante's reins, on account of the three thousand and odd thou art to give thyself for the disenchantment of Dulcinea.
>
> (De Cervantes, 1605/1615, p. 744)

Induced by the sadistic regime that they have just left, this "wild thought" (Bion, 1997), literally a thought "without a thinker", continues to emit its radioactive fallout and will soon manifest itself as insane aggression aimed at Sancho. Dulcinea is indeed in danger. The source of Cervantean inspiration can dry up at any moment, as long as he has not finished writing the book we are now reading.

When the author's torment over the highjacking of his work by learned brutes takes the form of a bullfight into which he sends his son without any warning, it is no wonder that the latter contemplates ending his life. Like children entrusted with caring for their parents without knowing what had wounded them, Don Quixote has no idea of the barbarities inflicted on his father by the forger Avellaneda.

Revealing cut-out history

Still unaware of the true objective of his third sally, the knight was to be informed of it the next day at the inn. Again, the author points out, "Don Quixote called it so, contrary to his usual practice of calling all inns castles" (De Cervantes, 1605/1615, p. 744). Cervantes has been repeating this formula each time the heroes arrived at new lodgings. If the reader is still unaware of the changes in Don Quixote's character, he must be a dolt.

Now, the megalomaniac is the innkeeper, who takes himself for a great chef running a four-star restaurant. Once he is brought back to his actual menu of cow heels and calves' feet, he goes off to prepare his guests' supper. In the meanwhile, Don Quixote overhears two voices in the room next to his own, talking about the "Second Part of Don Quixote of La Mancha", calling it an "absurd stuff" (De Cervantes, 1605/1615, p. 745). Worst of all, he hears that "Don Quixote [is] now cured of his love for Dulcinea del Toboso".

The real protagonist protests loudly through the partition that "the peerless Dulcinea del Toboso [cannot] be forgotten, nor can forgetfulness have a place in Don Quixote".

The truth, *aletheia*—which defies Lethe, the river of forgetfulness—was indeed what constituted the central stake of the First Part of *Don Quixote*. When Sancho confirms his master's identity, the two gentlemen burst into Don Quixote's room and recognise him at once: "Your appearance cannot leave any question as to your name, nor can your name fail to identify your appearance." These words attest that he is "the real Don Quixote de la Mancha", and at the same time inform him of the hijacking of his identity by Avellaneda, "who has sought to usurp your name and bring to naught your achievements" (De Cervantes, 1605/1615, p. 746).

They have concrete proof, in black and white, in the book that they present to him. After examining it briefly, Don Quixote discovers in it "three things [...] that deserve to be censured": some insulting remarks about Cervantes in the Prologue, the Aragonese language which sometimes dispenses with articles, and third, the fact that Teresa Panza is wrongly named Mari Gutierrez, while her husband is described as "a heavy feeder and a fool" (De Cervantes, 1605/1615, p. 746).

Foreseeing legislature for the protection of literary property—only introduced by Beaumarchais in France in 1777—the traveller suggests that "an order should be issued that no one should have the presumption to deal with anything relating to Don Quixote, save his original author Cide Hamete" (De Cervantes, 1605/1615, pp. 747–748).

While Sancho stays behind to feast on the stew concocted by the landlord, the knight accepts the travellers' invitation to share their supper, prepared by their own cook. But he refuses to read any more of the forger's book, so as not to give its author the occasion to flatter himself, but above all, he explains, because "our thoughts, and still more our eyes, should keep themselves aloof from what is obscene and filthy" (De Cervantes, 1605/1615, p. 748).

Of course, Dulcinea is the prime target of obscenity; she is suspected of being pregnant through the fault of the knight, and of being deeply disturbed by his feelings for her. Don Quixote confides in his hosts that it causes him great suffering to see her transformed into a country wench by an enchantment. They wonder if they should place him on the side of wisdom or folly. Apparently, they decide to adopt the definition of philosophical madness that Giordano Bruno applied to himself: "the madman is one whose knowledge does not conform to the common rule, for he aims higher, having greater intelligence" (Bruno, 1585).

Now, Don Quixote has had confirmation that the mission of his third sally has nothing to do with that of the first two. At the same time, he is shaken by this revelation. When children learn, at some point, about falsehoods concerning their identity, through letters or diaries found in an attic, or from comments made by a random visitor, the shock is hard to take. Like the hero, they feel betrayed and treated as if they are superfluous: "Let him who will paint me, but let him not abuse me; for patience will often break down when they heap insults upon it" (Bruno, 1585).

To expose the forgery, the only thing the knight can do is not follow the itinerary established by Avellaneda and by Carrasco (De Cervantes,

1605/1615, p. 414). "I will not set foot in Saragossa"—where the bachelor was urging him to take part in the jousting competition held on Saint George's Day—"and [...] I shall expose to the world the lie of this new history writer, and people will see that I am not the Don Quixote he speaks of".

The knight welcomes Don Jeronimo's suggestion that he participate instead in jousts held in Barcelona, especially since neither he nor Sancho have ever seen the sea. That beats everything, since we're talking about the son of a hero of naval battles, who is busy writing about adventures at sea in his *Trials of Persiles and Sigismunda* (1617).

Attack of madness

For six days following the shocking discovery made by Don Quixote, "nothing worthy of being recorded" happens, according to Cide Hamete. But when night comes after the seventh day, while he and Sancho are resting, like God, in a thicket of oak trees, Don Quixote has an attack of madness.

The wild man, medieval incarnation of madness, awakens with the fury accumulated during the events of the previous episode. The actual attacks on his life are real. The agency of the Lady of his thoughts, compromised by Sancho in Toboso, must be reaffirmed. Now, a manic episode is acted out when Don Quixote cannot sleep; the image of Dulcinea transformed into a country wench "[roams] in fancy to and fro through all sorts of places" (De Cervantes, 1605/1615, p. 749). The trace of the perverse scenario is not easy to erase.

Back to Freud's primary process in which words are things and things are words: when the given word does not hold, metaphors are enacted literally. The sinister vision of Merlin ordering Sancho to give himself three thousand lashes is quasi-hallucinatory. Divided between his loyalty to Dulcinea and to his squire, Don Quixote decides to cut the Gordian knot, like Alexander the Great did: "[what] if I scourge Sancho against his will ..."

The phrase "To cut comes to the same things as to untie" impels him to untie, literally, the points of Sancho's breeches, to flog his bare buttocks. The squire wakes up and cries out: "What is this? Who is touching me and untrussing me?"

Standing above him, his master, distraught but determined, attempts to explain his mad design: "Dulcinea is perishing, thou art living on regardless, I am dying of hope deferred; therefore untruss thyself with a good will, for mine it is, here, in this retired spot, to give thee at least two thousand lashes" (De Cervantes, 1605/1615, p. 750).

In the face of such ruthless logic, Sancho understands at once that there is no use arguing, nor trying to prove that the lashes "must be voluntary". Better act right away. When his master tried to untie the points of his breeches, Sancho got up suddenly, and grappled with him: "he gripped him with all his might in his arms, giving him a trip with the heel stretched him on the ground on his back, and pressing on his right knee on his chest held his hands in his own, so that he could neither move nor breathe" (De Cervantes, 1605/1615, p. 750).

Pinned to the ground, the knight is outraged—let's not forget the feudal tradition—that Sancho dares to "revolt against [his] master and natural lord". Unhesitatingly, the squire invokes the right to disobey orders when the superior has lost his head: "I neither put down king, nor set up king, […] I only stand up for myself who am my own lord."

This demonstrates that such a crisis can recede when a subject is able to stand up as "other", to assert his rights simply, without hatred. Indeed, the incident ends with Sancho asking the knight to promise not to behave like this again. Knowing his master, he trusts him to keep his promise. Their alliance is strengthened and Don Quixote calms down: "[He] swore by the life of his thoughts not to touch so much as a hair of his garments, and to leave him entirely free and to his own discretion to whip himself whenever he pleased" (De Cervantes, 1605/1615, p. 750).

Going off to sleep undisturbed at the foot of a tree some distance away, Sancho "felt something touch his head, and putting up his hands encountered somebody's two feet …". He screamed: a hanged man!

Ballad of the hanged (Villon)

Don Quixote surmises that they are not far from Barcelona, since Catalonia is overrun by bandits and the authorities "are wont to hang them up by twenties and thirties when they catch them" (De Cervantes, 1605/1615, p. 751).

This cannot fail to bring to mind the French folk song "La Complainte de Mandrin", about the famous bandit Louis Mandrin, executed in 1755.

> We were twenty or thirty, outlaws in a band,
> All dressed in white, hear what I say,
> Dressed in white like merchants.

Indeed, at dawn, "upward of forty living [outlaws] all of a sudden surrounded" the knight and squire. Unarmed, Don Quixote nods at them and waits proudly, arms folded and head bowed, while they take everything Dapple carries, but not the money, which Sancho had in a girdle that he wore around his body. Fortunately, their captain arrives and interrupts the looting.

A Pyrenean version of Mandrin from the Alps, roaming the Dauphiné region, this very handsome gunman, about thirty-five, "strongly built, above the middle height, of stern aspect and swarthy complexion" (De Cervantes, 1605/1615, p. 751), is not some brutal highwayman, but a celebrated historical figure: Roque Guinart, as famous as Gines de Passamonte, but much less villainous. In fact, he ended his life where Cervantes had started his military career, in the Spanish troops in Naples, after receiving a royal pardon.

The two men know each other by reputation, and hold each other in mutual respect. Although he has never taken Don Quixote's adventures seriously, the great Roque notices the knight's sadness and strives to fight it, like a brother-in-arms. They converse on an equal footing. After his recent disappointment, the knight is strongly tempted by their lawless life, not so different from his own. The bandit agrees: is it not true that one way to treat trauma is to take the law into one's own hands, when there is no other justice to be had? He admits that he is "by nature tender-hearted and kindly, but [...] the desire to revenge [himself] for a wrong [...] so overturns all [his] better impulses that [he keeps] on in his way of life" (De Cervantes, 1605/1615, p. 755).

Don Quixote too has chosen a life of errantry: "it is my duty, according to the rule of knight-errantry which I profess, to be always on the alert and at all times my own sentinel".

The life of the outlaws, which the knight will share for three days and three nights, is, like his own, full of "strange adventures, strange incidents, and all full of danger. [...] They slept standing, breaking their slumbers to shift from place to place" (De Cervantes, 1605/1615, pp. 755, 759). Like Don Quixote, they valued justice. When the time came to share the bounty, Roque "made shares for the whole band so equitably and carefully, that in no case did he exceed or fall short of strict distributive justice". In addition, his sense of honour had earned him a reputation of generosity, somewhat like a Catalan Robin Hood.

In fact, the events that follow confirm this reputation, when a group of travellers is held up. The members of the group represent all three traditional segments of society: the military, the nobility, and pilgrims. Some are travelling to Naples, others to Rome. The booty taken from them is considerable. After creating an interval of suspense, Roque restores their possessions in a most chivalrous manner, asking only that they pay a fee for safe passage to Barcelona: "for I have no intention of doing injury to soldiers, or to any woman, especially one of quality" (De Cervantes, 1605/1615, p. 757).

What could be more noble? Don Quixote is delighted. The only thing missing is the defence of virgins; but just then such a damsel makes a well-timed entrance, at a furious pace.

Guerrillera

Claudia Jeronima makes her appearance attired like a splendid young guerrilero: "tight-fitting polished boots, with a hat looped in the Waloon fashion, gilt spurs, dagger and sword, and in his hand a musketoon, and a pair of pistols at his waist" (De Cervantes, 1605/1615, p. 752)—the picture is complete. She asks the bandit riding up and down along the border—as a spy, as a robber, and sometimes as a smuggler of Huguenots—to help her cross in the opposite direction, because she has just committed a crime of passion. Don Quixote is stunned by the fair maiden's request to the valiant Roque, delivered in the purest knightly rhetoric.

Her story constitutes a reversal of the situation of Lucinda enamoured with Cardenio, and Quitterie in love with Basile, both of them forced to marry against their will. Claudia loves Don Vicente and, being a hotheaded girl, she fires a musket at him, hitting him in the chest, because she has heard rumours that he is about to marry another. Don Quixote offers to defend her, and Sancho praises his master's talent as a matchmaker, citing his success in the case of the duena's daughter.

However, Cervantes foresees the possibility that future readers may imitate Don Quixote as a way of escaping the law. Therefore, he makes things quite clear. His hero must not be used to justify anything and everything. First, a distinction must be made between different kinds of damsels. Clearly, those who are scatterbrained—the duena's daughter, Camilla, in the story of the Ill-Advised Curiosity (De Cervantes, 1605/1615, p. 233), or this Geronima—exasperate him, perhaps because of the mischief his own daughter Isabel gets into; they should all be sent to a convent, he thinks.

The fair Claudia's elegant costume does not compensate for her bad judgement, which caused the death of an innocent man. When Roque took her back to the wounded Don Vicente, the young man denied the false rumours her jealousy had inflated, asked her to press his hands and take him for her husband, and took his last breath.

The tragedy to which he was a powerless witness drew tears from the outlaw's eyes, "unused as they were to shed them on any occasion" (De Cervantes, 1605/1615, p. 754), but he said not a word. Claudia herself stopped playing the role of a *desperada* and, in real despair, "would not [...] allow him to accompany her; and thanking him for his offers as well as she could, took leave of him in tears". While Roque is unable to speak, Don Quixote, mounted on Rocinante, delivers a harangue to his men, "[urging] them to give up a mode of life so full of peril, as well to the soul as to the body".

Besides, he equal distribution of the booty is not respected out of concern for justice, but out of fear of violence, because the possibility of murder is never far off: "If this scrupulous exactness were not observed with these fellows there would be no living with them", their leader had told Don Quixote (De Cervantes, 1605/1615, p. 755).

The point is proven on the spot. When Sancho speaks of "thieves", thus showing disrespect to the outlaws, one of them almost breaks his head with his harquebus. Similarly, Celestina was killed by Calisto's servants, who were themselves condemned to public execution. Told that they are threatened with the same fate, Guinart's accomplices appear too dull-witted to care: "but as most of them were Gascons, rough lawless fellows, [the knight's] speech did not make much impression on them" (De Cervantes, 1605/1615, p. 754).

Don Quixote then turns to their captain, since they have already established easy transference. When Roque confesses that the life he has chosen is contrary to his nature, Don Quixote insists on psychoanalysing him: "Señor Roque, the beginning of health lies in knowing the disease and in the sick man's willingness to take the medicines which the physician prescribes" (De Cervantes, 1605/1615, p. 756).

Therapy seems possible. Given the charm, spirit, intelligence, and talents of the potential patient, all that's needed is a series of regular sessions: "medicines [...] cure gradually, and not of a sudden or by a miracle [...]. Come with me, and I will show you how to become a knight-errant".

Roque laughed. In truth, sparing the group of travellers was just a way of impressing Don Quixote, for he had not yet decided to give up this way of life. In addition, he was on good terms with those who governed the region: the knight understood that his affairs were going well, and stopped giving him advice.

This opponent of the established order needs his band of accomplices, although he fears them as much as they fear him. "Roque passed his nights in some place or other apart from his men, that they might not know where he was, for [...] he did not venture to trust anyone, afraid that his own men would kill him or deliver him up to the authorities" (De Cervantes, 1605/1615, p. 759).

The psychoanalysis of trauma seems antithetical to criminal systems. Roque laughs at Don Quixote's suggestion, but magnanimously escorts him to the outskirts of Barcelona, since he finds him to be "the drollest and wisest man in the world".

He cannot place the knight in any psychiatric category, nor associate him with any political affiliation. He does not belong to any clan: neither that of the nobility, which includes Roque's friends, nor that of his enemies. Party boundaries do not apply, "because the crazes and shrewd sayings of Don Quixote and the humors of his squire Sancho Panza could not help giving general pleasure to all the world" (De Cervantes, 1605/1615, p. 758).

Cervantes' political problem, eighty pages before the end of the novel, is how to bring his "supersonic" son into a world where addiction, predation, cheating, and pretence are part of the normal social link. The fall will be hard, especially after the marvellous vacation the author provided for his son on the shores of the Mediterranean. It was there that everything began for him forty years earlier, when he was captured by pirates off the Costa Brava. The knight's arrival in the city is greeted with unexpected enthusiasm.

Thalassa!

The date is 21 June: "At length, by unfrequented roads, short cuts, and secret paths [...] they reached the strand on Saint John's Eve during the night." The dawn brightened the sky to welcome the hero. A din of clarions, drums, and bells was heard, and "the sun […] with a face broader than a buckler began to rise" (De Cervantes, 1605/1615, p. 759).

The dazzling emergence of the Sun god presides over their first glimpse of the sea:

> Don Quixote and Sancho gazed all around them; they beheld the sea, a sight until then unseen by them; it struck them as exceedingly spacious and broad, much more so than the lakes of Ruidera […]. They saw the galleys along the beach, […] lowering their awnings, […] decked with streamers and pennons that trembled in the breeze […], while on board the bugles, trumpets, and clarions were sounding,
>
> (De Cervantes, 1605/1615, p. 758)

to create a naval show by keeping up ceaseless artillery fire against the cannons on the walls and forts of the city: "The bright sea, smiling earth, the clear air—though at times darkened by the smoke of the guns—all seemed to fill the whole multitude with unexpected delight" (De Cervantes, 1605/1615, p. 759).

The entrance of Don Quixote on the stage of this festive period of the zodiac signals the return of the spirit of life after the crossing of deadly zones. His arrival is greeted with cheers by a small troop of horsemen in livery. One of them addressed him directly, saying the words he wanted to hear:

> Welcome to our city, mirror, beacon, star and cynosure of all knight-errantry […]! Welcome, I say, valiant Don Quixote of La Mancha; not the false, the fictitious, the apocryphal, that these latter days have offered us in lying histories, but the true, the legitimate, the real one that Cide Hamete Benengeli, flower of historians, has described to us!
>
> (De Cervantes, 1605/1615, p. 760)

This is the least Cervantes can do for his son, through the intervention of the great Roque, whose friend "Don Antonio Moreno […], a gentleman of wealth and intelligence", to whose house the heroes are led ceremoniously. Don Antonio is fond of amusements, but contrary to the ducal court, "he set about devising modes of making [Don Quixote] exhibit his mad points in some harmless fashion; for jests that give pain are no jests, and no sport is worth anything if it hurts another" (De Cervantes, 1605/1615, p. 762).

Now that he is reunited with this old child of his who has conducted commando attacks on "our depraved era", Cervantes wants him to enjoy himself: "Some of Don Antonio's friends dined with him that day, and all showed honor to Don Quixote and treated him as a knight-errant, and he becoming puffed up and exalted in consequence could not contain himself for satisfaction" (De Cervantes, 1605/1615, p. 762).

The gentleman is determined to be an excellent host and to provide strolls, dancing, the discovery of a printing office, and, to top everything off, a ride on a galley. The visit of the mansion starts with a cabinet of curiosities where Don Antonio keeps an automaton, a talking head "after the fashion of the busts of Roman emperors". A forerunner of the telephone, this curious contrivance is one of many avant-garde devices described in the novel:

> [it] was hollow throughout, as was the table, [...] and the whole was in communication with another room underneath the chamber in which the head stood. [...] In the room below [...] was placed the person who was to answer, with his mouth to the tube, and the voice, as in an ear trumpet, passed from above downwards, and from below upwards; it was impossible, thus, to detect the trick.
>
> (De Cervantes, 1605/1615, p. 768)

For those who questioned the head, the device acted like the "*che vuoi?*" in Jacques Cazotte's *The Devil in Love* (1772), referring each questioner back to his own desire. Sancho learns what he already knows; the head tells him: "Thou shalt govern in thy house [when] thou shalt cease to be a squire." As for Don Quixote, he is told: "The disenchantment of Dulcinea will attain its due consummation."

Then, Don Quixote was taken for a stroll through the city, with a parchment bearing his name stitched to his overcoat, and he soon became the object of mockery. A Castilian passer-by hurled insults at him, in a manner reminiscent of the furious ecclesiastic at the ducal castle: "Get thee home, blockhead, and see after thy affairs, and thy wife and children."

But whereas the duchess would have prolonged the humiliation, Don Antonio removes the parchment to prevent any more incidents of this kind. Cervantes also considers that it is time to end the farce. His son deserves to retire peacefully. It is time to set Dulcinea's disenchantment in motion, not in order for Don Quixote to return to his old self, but because she is no longer needed. We have gone beyond the stage where the knight, spurred on by the violent wind of reviviscences, is charged with the mission of inscribing the adventures of the former slave and soldier. As for the present fight against his father's literary enemies, it will soon come to an end. Enough is enough!

A dancing party given in the evening resulted in such exertion that the knight's puppet-like state was shaken off for good: "[Two ladies] of a mischievous and frolicsome turn [...] tired him down, not only in body but in spirit." Too much is too much. "Don Quixote [...], long, lank, lean, and yellow, his garments clinging tight to him, ungainly, and above all anything but agile" let himself drop to the floor and "sat down [...] in the middle of the room, tired out and broken down by all this exertion in the dance", and repelled the flirtatious ladies. It is clear that an inner spring is broken. The soul of the dancing puppet—the ancestor of the puppet in Heinrich von Kleist's essay "The Puppet Theatre" (1810, p. 411) whose movements are so natural because it doesn't need to put on airs—has finished healing his father's traumas. The marionette can now assume human form.

A safe haven

Don Antonio's "large and stately" house is in fact a safe haven where Don Quixote can become himself again, and wander alone wherever he likes, without following a cultural programme. Small wonder that his meanderings take him to the door of a printing house: "he was vastly pleased, for until then he had never seen a printing office, and he was curious to know what it was like" (De Cervantes, 1605/1615, p. 768). Once inside, he had the opportunity to speak to an author who was supervising the printing of a translation, and to prove the inadequacy of translations from Italian to Castilian (De Cervantes, 1605/1615, p. 769), with the exception of a pastoral tragicomedy, and Torquato Tasso's *Aminta*.

The discussion gets heated when it broaches intellectual pirates who highjack a work and the network of its readers. Publishers, called booksellers at that time, are severely criticised, especially those who make the author feel they are "doing [him] a favor" (De Cervantes, 1605/1615, p. 770). Don Quixote's interlocutor concludes his diatribe with this heart-felt avowal: "I want to make money, without which reputation is not worth a cent."

A word to the wise! After this indictment, the reader is not surprised to find that one of the books being corrected in the printing office is the fake *Second Part of the Ingenious Gentleman Don Quixote of La Mancha*, which the knight attacks mercilessly: "I have heard of this book already, and verily and on my conscience I thought it had been by this time burned to ashes as a meddlesome intruder; but its Martinmas will come as it does to every pig" (De Cervantes, 1605/1615, p. 770).

So far, so good. Still, before putting an end to his hero's life, as he announced in the Prologue, Cervantes must rectify an important omission. The initial event, the source of all the knight's adventures, is absent from the first novel. Even the most careful reader will fail to find the least reference to the capture of Miguel and his brother Rodrigo by Ottoman pirates. This forgetfulness—unconscious slip, or splitting off—shall be set right at once.

In fact, the highpoint of the second novel is an enactment of the original scene, in the grandiose style of a Hollywood superproduction. To get an idea of what it might have been like, one can visit, at the Barcelona Naval Museum, the reconstruction of Juan of Austria's galley—which emerged victorious from the battle of Lepante—with special effects embodying the rowers sweating at their benches. On the walls, paintings and mosaics from Cervantes' era depict for the reader scenes similar to the naval show, and celebrations of the summer solstice. As for Sancho, he sees himself acting as captain in command: "though, as has been said, he hated being a governor, still he had a longing to be giving orders and finding himself obeyed once more; this is the misfortune that being in authority, even in jest, brings with it" (De Cervantes, 1605/1615, p. 771).

Here, Cervantes speaks in his own name as well, for he has trouble letting go of the reins of his novel. He is in charge and arranges for us to enjoy a naval parade and witness a mock attack by pirates. But the show experienced in reality bears the mark of authenticity. As Don Quixote told the corrector of the *Second Part*, forgers have no access to this truth: "for fictions have the more merit and charm about them the more nearly they approach the truth [...]; and true stories, the truer they are the better they are".

Apotheosis: all aboard!

Let us imagine the galleys in the port of Barcelona, where Don Antonio now took Don Quixote. In honour of his son, Cervantes, the seafarer, has put on a royal display:

> all the galleys struck their awnings and the clarions rang out. A skiff covered with red carpets and cushions of crimson velvet was immediately lowered into the water, and as Don Quixote stepped on board of it, the leading galley fired her gangway gun, and the other galleys did the same.
>
> (De Cervantes, 1605/1615, p. 771)

The tribute paid to the knight, "delighted beyond measure with such a lordly reception", was enacted according to the state-of-the-art rules of maritime and theatrical tradition. Sancho was to play the fool when the aftermost rower "[hoisted] him up in his arms, and the whole crew [...], proceeded to pass him on, whirling him along from hand to hand, and from bench to bench", very quickly from starboard to port. When the galley was laying anchor, and the boatswain was laying lashes on the shoulders of the men with his whip, Don Quixote told Sancho to take advantage of the opportunity and have himself whipped, for "[amid] the pain and sufferings of so many you would not feel your own much".

The reference to hell, "or at least purgatory", inflicted on the galley crew provides a perfect transition to the real capture of a Turkish vessel, similar to the capture of the *El Sol*, the galley carrying Miguel and his brother Rodrigo in 1575 off the Catalan shores. Cervantes has not forgotten his kidnapping at the age of twenty-eight. His citations for bravery and the letters to the king found on him raised his ransom so much that the course of his life was altered forever!

Nearly forty years later, the crewman on watch cries out that the Montjui watchtower overlooking Barcelona "signals that there is an oared vessel off the coast to the west". The chase is on: "The three other [vessels] immediately came alongside the chief galley to receive their orders", and put out to sea at a furious pace. The brigantine "judged to be one of fourteen or fifteen banks, went about with the object and in the hope of making her escape by her speed". But the chief galley is one of the fastest vessels on the Mediterranean and the Moorish captain is soon ready to surrender.

At that moment, "two Toraquis, that is to say two Turks, both drunken", kill two sailors on the chief galley. There will be no mercy! "the general swore that he would not leave one of those he found on board the vessel alive, [and] he bore down furiously upon her". The chase continues; the brigantine slips away "by sailing and rowing", but the galley catches up with it and the Spanish sailors overrun it. The whole crew is taken alive. The four galleys weigh anchor near the shore. The viceroy arrives on a jolly-boat. A space is cleared for the hanging of the Turkish crew, "the captain and the rest of the men […] about six-and-thirty in number, all smart fellows", before a crowd of onlookers gathered on the shore" (De Cervantes, 1605/1615, p. 773).

Dramatic twist

The captain of the brigantine, a handsome youth not yet twenty, speaks Castilian. He brings to mind the magnificent Billy Bud Sailor (Melville, 1891), hung from the highest yardarm two centuries later, after being ambushed by a scoundrel.

Written just before Melville's death, the story also recounts the author's own seafaring adventures. Now is a good time to sing a sea shanty:

> Let us sing, to pass the time,
> The joyful loves of a maiden
> Who, disguised as a sailor,
> Boarded the vessel in haste.
> As soon as she was engaged
> She embarked upon the ship,
> Quickly donned a sailor suit
> And embarked upon the ship.

With the rope already around his neck, the young captain reveals his identity:

> I am neither Turk, nor Moor, nor renegade.
> —What art thou then? said the viceroy.
> —A Christian woman, replied the youth.
>
> (De Cervantes, 1605/1615, p. 774)

To top it all off, she was born of Morisco parents. When the Moors were being ousted from Spain, she was taken to Barbary against her will by two of her uncles; her suitor, the young nobleman Gaspar Gregorio, who fortunately speaks Arabic, has followed her. On her advice, he disguised himself as a woman, "for among those barbarous Turks a fair youth is more esteemed than a woman, be she ever so beautiful" (De Cervantes, 1605/1615, p. 775).

She dons her own disguise on orders from the dey of Algiers, who sends her back to her village in Spain to recover the treasure left buried there by her father, on a vessel with Turks, Moors, and a renegade. In the meantime, her suitor is about to be sent off as a present to the Grand Signor in Constantinople, where Cervantes would have been taken had his ransom not been paid a day earlier. Then, all trace of him would have been lost. One of those listening to her story, a pilgrim who had come aboard with the viceroy, cried out: "O Ana Felix, my unhappy daughter, I am thy father Ricote, come back to look for thee, unable to live without thee, my soul that thou art!"

Sancho confirms his neighbour's identity. The captain decides to reduce the number of Turks to be hanged, limiting it to the two men responsible for the incident. In the end, the viceroy obtains a pardon for them. The scenario of the return of the hostages may be cliché, but it still applies today. A decision is made to send to Algiers the renegade entrusted with the young girl, to bring back her captive lover; he is to set off in a six-bench vessel manned by Christian rowers. Ricote promises to pay their ransom, should they be captured.

Here, Cervantes introduces an important "character": *The Mediterranean and the Mediterranean World in the Age of Philip II*, as it is portrayed by Fernand Braudel (1949), who wrote this work while a prisoner of war in the Second World War. Indeed, History enters the scene, on both sides of the *Mare Nostrum*, overturning oppositions: a girl transformed into a boy, and the other way around, a Christian changed into a Muslim, and vice versa, Spaniards boarding a brigantine from Algiers, as the reverse of the boarding of Cervantes' galley by the Ottomans.

In fact, Don Quixote is so eager to participate in Don Gregorio's rescue and to visit Algiers, that he is ready to leap over to the other shore at a moment's notice. He offers "to land himself with arms and horse in Barbary", as Don Gaiferos did to rescue his wife Melisandra, but Sancho is there to remind him of the laws of geography: "Remember, your worship, Señor Don Gaiferos carried off his wife from the mainland, and took her to France by land, but in this case [...], there's the sea between" (De Cervantes, 1605/1615, p. 778).

"No matter", his master answers, unabashed, that courage conquers all: "There's a remedy for everything except death."

The renegade is sent off to rescue Don Gregorio, and Don Antonio promises that in case he fails, he will send the great Don Quixote to Barbary.

In the meantime, before the young suitor is brought back, the knight undergoes a spiritual transformation. He must now discard everything that counts for him. Does this mean, as the saying goes, that he will suffer a "real" depression? That would amount to confusing entering madness with emerging from it. In fact, while both take the form of a crisis, they lead in different directions: one brings about the stopping of time, while the other sets arrested time in motion, as is the case in this instance. Alchemy is at work, producing one last refinement of the knight's psyche.

Nunc dimittis

To bring his novel and his life to an end, Cervantes chooses the tones of Ronsard's "Derniers vers" (Final Song) (2002, p. 267):

> One must leave houses and orchards and gardens,
> Tableware and jars engraved by craftsmen,
> And sing of one's burial like the swan
> Who sings before his passing on Turkish shores.
> It's done, my destiny's fulfilled,
> I've lived and made my name into renown,
> My pen flies to the sky to be some sign,
> Far from earthly charms that deceive the most enlightened.

In 1917, infantrymen sang their own "Final Song"—*La Chanson de Craonne,* where thousands died—during the offensive of the French Army on the Chemin des Dames:

> Good-bye to life, good-bye to love, good-bye to all the women,
> It's all over now, we've had it for good with this awful war.
> It's in Craonne upon the plateau that we must end our lives.

"Goodbye, humor, goodbye, wit; goodbye merry friends; for I am dying and hope to see you soon, happy in the life to come! " (De Cervantes, 1617, p. 20).

With these words, written three days before his death in 1616, Cervantes ended the Prologue to *The Trials of Persiles and Sigismunda* (1617). But before that, he had written Don Quixote's farewell to Dulcinea, once his mission had been accomplished. The episode of the capture by Barbary pirates appeared in print in 1614, just as the battles of Lepanto and La Goulette (De Cervantes, 1605/1615, Vol. I, chapters XXXIX to XLI) were described in the first novel, along with the bagnios of Algiers.

Still, Cervantes asks himself, how is he to make the knight understand that Dulcinea, who has always been his muse, has now fulfilled her purpose? She needs a superb exit, so he sets up nothing less than a rendez-vous of the sun with the moon, like in the Charles Trenet song:

> The sun has a date with the moon,
> But the moon is not there and the sun waits for her.

But, in this instance, the full moon is there to meet the sun at his solstice. The astrological setting is magnificent, and the meeting of the two takes the form of a clash. A knight with a shining moon painted on his shield came to meet Don Quixote one morning when he "went out for a stroll [...] arrayed in full armor". He approached, saying he was the Knight of the White Moon, and challenged Don Quixote to acknowledge "that my lady, let her be who she may, is incomparably fairer than thy Dulcinea del Toboso". The conditions are simple and clear. "If thou fightest and I vanquish thee, I demand no other satisfaction than that, laying aside arms and abstaining from going in quest of adventures, thou withdraw and betake thyself to thine own village for the space of a year, [...] for the increase of thy substance and the salvation of thy soul" (De Cervantes, 1605/1615, p. 779). If it should be Don Quixote who vanquishes the knight, the latter places his head at Don Quixote's mercy, and grants him his arms and his horse as spoils.

Don Quixote takes up the challenge. The viceroy is informed of the confrontation and hurries to the beach with Don Antonio and other gentlemen, to try to prevent this unexpected duel. Impossible! The time has come for Don Quixote to give up Dulcinea.

Will Cervantes betray his hero and collaborate with his son's enemies, as was the case at the end of the first novel? All the signs are there, for the duel is quickly over.

Dulcinea's disenchantment

The two knights took the necessary distance. The charge of the White Moon was swifter and met Don Quixote after two-thirds of the course, his lance held high. He hit him with such violence that Don Quixote and Rocinante were hurled to the ground, then lept on top of him, placing the lance over his helmet. Don Quixote lifted his visor and conceded defeat "in a weak feeble voice as if he were speaking out of a tomb" (De Cervantes, 1605/1615, p. 780). He reaffirmed his faith in Dulcinea, asked his adversary to drive his lance home and put an end to a life that had lost all meaning. Finally, he agreed to retire to his village, "so long as nothing in prejudice of Dulcinea was demanded of him" (De Cervantes, 1605/1615, p. 780).

Onlookers and readers are left dejected after witnessing this scene. Sancho, especially, is woebegone, and thinking "that the whole business was a dream". As for Don Antonio, he was charged with clearing up the mystery by following the Knight of the White Moon to his hostel in the city.

The enigmatic character makes no attempt to conceal his true identity. He is, of course, the bachelor Sanson Carrasco, whose actions are carried out so that Don Quixote "might be cured" (De Cervantes, 1605/1615, p. 782), with the best medical intentions, since "his chance of recovery lay in quiet". But the reader, who remembers events of which the Catalan gentleman is unaware, understands that the student has just taken revenge for the defeat he suffered three months earlier, in the spring, when he presented himself under the guise of Knight of the Mirrors. Hate disguised as concern for the other's well-being requires secrecy, if the plan is to succeed. "I implore you not to betray me, or tell Don Quixote who I am; so that my honest endeavors may be successful, and that a man of excellent wits—were he only rid of the fooleries of chivalry—may get them back again" (De Cervantes, 1605/1615, p. 782).

Recognising the habits of the ducal castle, the reader is likely thinking: "We have come all this way to end up like this!" We could almost feel angry with Cervantes for causing us to tumble, along with our beloved hero, who is now being lifted up, "pale and bathed with sweat". Don Antonio takes it upon himself to express our disappointment to the student, more elegantly than we could have done:

> O señor, may God forgive you the wrong you have done the whole world in trying to bring the most amusing madman in it back to his senses [...]; and if it were not uncharitable, I would say may Don Quixote never be cured, for by his recovery we lose not only his own drolleries, but his squire Sancho Panza's too, any one of which is enough to turn melancholy itself into merriment. However, I'll hold my peace and say nothing to him, and we'll see whether I am right in my suspicion that Señor Carrasco's efforts will be fruitless.
>
> (De Cervantes, 1605/1615, p. 782)

Now, the puzzled reader no longer knows what to think, since the treatment recommended by the caregivers consists, once again, of rest, pseudo-therapeutic activity, strolls, meals, naps, pseudo-work, rest, and, above all, no connection with history—one's own story caught up in History. Like Don Antonio, the reader hopes wholeheartedly that "Señor Carrasco's efforts" and his daft psychodrama "will be fruitless".

We are still children when the show is over and the curtain falls. One lucky day, after standing in line for a long while outside the Comédie-Française in Paris, the seats in the President's box were offered for sale to the public at the last minute, for Molière's play *The Would-Be Gentleman*, which was sold out. We had our elder son with us, who was six, and was coming to a real theatre for the first time, to see the famous play staged by Jean Le Poulain. The comedy-ballet, with music composed by Jean-Baptiste Lully, kept him spellbound, but at the end of the performance the spell was abruptly broken by the director himself.

After Monsieur Jourdain was promoted to the status of Mamamouchi, the stage set collapsed noisily and the Gentleman, left on a bare stage, made his exit arm in arm with his wife, a comforting bottle of wine in his hand. Enthusiastic applause rose from the crowd, punctured by the piercing scream of a wounded animal. Our son, who had sat silently through the performance, was crying noisily, refusing to move, while the crowd was walking out, throwing disapproving glances in the direction of the President's box.

From manipulation to masterpiece

Don Quixote, just as immobile, "[kept] to his bed six days, dejected, melancholy, moody and out of sorts, brooding over the unhappy event of his defeat". As usual, Sancho tried to raise his spirits: "Hold up your head, señor, and be of good cheer if you can, and give thanks to heaven that if you have had a tumble to the ground you have not come off with a broken rib [...]; rightly looked at, it is I that am the greater loser" (De Cervantes, 1605/1615, p. 783).

In the meantime, the lovers have been reunited. The renegade's expedition has brought Don Gregorio back to Ricote's daughter. "They did not embrace each other, for where there is deep love there will never be overwhelming boldness" (De Cervantes, 1605/1615, p. 784). Like at the end of the first novel, Don Quixote is absent from the scene enacting the success of an enterprise indirectly brought about through his efforts. But he has blazed a new path—as mountaineers say when they name a trail after the first man who climbed it.

The Quixotic trail opens a passage into the political manoeuvres of the time. The knight's absence was already clearly indicated when Lucinda and Cardenio, and Dorothea and her seducer, Don Fernando, were reunited. Still, the very ones who would never have seen each other again without his intervention were more than willing to collaborate in his being caged up. The reader fears the worst, since experience has shown that traumatised fathers, like Cervantes, can sometimes be very hard on their children.

The "happy ending" scenario is similar to that of the first novel. Don Antonio will intercede on behalf of the Ricote family at the Court in the capital, to enable them to stay in Spain, despite the eagerness to banish the Moors shown by Don Bernardino de Velasco, whose "Argus eyes [were] ever on the watch lest one [...] should remain behind in concealment". And while the two lovers walk off into a future full of promise, Don Quixote and Sancho exit looking pitiful, like the Would-Be Gentleman with his wife, their backs to the spectators, on an empty stage. On the road again! "Don Quixote without his armor [...], and Sancho on foot, Dapple being loaded with the armor" (De Cervantes, 1605/1615, p. 785): the suspense is at its peak and the sadness infinite.

How will Cervantes' novel end after such a disheartening turn of events? The wise reader, whose spirits have been invigorated by ever-renewed energy up until now, is becoming discouraged. We are far from the Catalan apotheosis performed to our delight. As usual, Don Quixote assumes responsibility for his actions: "'each of us is the maker of his own Fortune'. I have been that of mine; but not with the proper amount of prudence" (De Cervantes, 1605/1615, p. 786).

Nevertheless, he is not about to lose all hope: "Forward then, Sancho my friend, let us go to keep the year of the novitiate in our own country, and in that seclusion we shall pick up fresh strength to return to the by me never-forgotten calling of arms" (De Cervantes, 1605/1615, p. 786).

What does Cervantes mean by this? Is Don Quixote's novitiate the one into which Cervantes entered, at the same period, before taking vows in the Tertiary Franciscan Order? Does the temporary renunciation accepted by Don Quixote correspond to the author's relinquishing of his hero like to a never-to-be-forgotten part of himself? We go back to square one, as always when the analysis of madness or trauma is almost accomplished. Yet the spot where Don Quixote fell clearly marks a point of no-return: "Here Troy was, here my ill luck, not my cowardice, robbed me of all the glory I had won; [...] here, in a word, fell my happiness never to rise again."

Cervantes makes his hero go through his previous adventures again at an accelerated pace, like in a cumulative song. Sancho's government, the defence of the duena, Altisidora's tricks, the fake Arcadia, Sancho's self-flogging, six hundred pigs instead of bulls, the castle of the duke and duchess, Altisidora (encore), the flogging (encore), the forger's book—are all revisited one by one. After this overview, the return to the village takes place in a radically different state of mind, for at every stage an alternative is found to the fatal "never more", as Poe would say.

What is left of our loves?

What is left of an analysis after multiple returns to square one, in a time that moves in circles, suggesting that there has been no progress? The question is crucial and the answer escapes quantification, for the signs of a subject's ability to escape destruction do not lend themselves to "evidence-based" description. Why do we agree to say that astrophysical phenomena are not reproducible, but refuse to say so about psychic phenomena? And why does the birth of a subject deserve less attention than the birth of a star?

Cervantes answers this question at the end of the novel, showing that the birth of a subject is inseparable from his downfall. The object of the knight's search is himself. Like Actaeon, the hunted hunter, he finds himself pinned to the ground by the Knight of the White Moon, and he goes over the different events that led up to this moment, recalling them with Sancho. At the conclusion of an analysis of madness and trauma, a new ability to judge has been acquired.

When Don Quixote and Sancho are asked to settle a dispute in a village during a festival, Sancho naturally offers to exercise his authority in judging the question. A fat man has challenged a thin man to run a race, not unlike the race between Carrasco's huge horse and Rocinante. The fat man wants to force his opponent to carry iron on his back to equalise their weights. Contrariwise, Sancho enjoins the fat man to trim some of his fat. The villagers are delighted with the verdict and decide to "let half the wager be spent in wine".

The most remarkable thing about this sentence is that the squire steps up to answer in his master's place. In the course of their adventures, Sancho has acquired openly recognised wisdom: "If the servant is so clever, what must the master be?" The villagers go on to comment that no one will be able to take it away from him, be they in positions obtained through favours, or graduates of the Salamanca university (De Cervantes, 1605/1615, p. 788). Sancho's judgement also reveals that his master's defeat in the duel was brought about unfairly, given that there was no referee to decide about the position of the sun and the disproportion between the two horses.

What is left of the daring feat which restored the duena's honour and that of her daughter? The unexpected encounter with the lackey Tosilos, on his way to deliver letters from the duke and duchess to the viceroy in Barcelona, seems to make the answer obvious. Nothing much. Perversion, once uncovered, unlashes violence—as it happened with André—as soon as those who revealed it have their backs turned. Tosilos was given a hundred lashes by the duke, the duena's daughter entered a convent, and the duena went back to Castile. But they had had a chance to refuse submitting to the prevailing order. What came of it was out of Don Quixote's control. Besides, he never used his generous deeds for self-promotion. He had enough to do just to deal with the paternal reviviscences crowding in upon him.

His adventures have left him not so much with a feeling of satisfaction, as with harassing questions. These thoughts went round and round in his head and "like flies on honey, [they] came crowding upon him and stinging him" (De Cervantes, 1605/1615, p. 790). Anyone who has ever been harassed by a bee determined to lead him away from the hive knows exactly how much insomnia resembles the buzzing of that insect. Altisidora is arousing regrets in Don Quixote's mind, about not giving her this or that: "[she] loved me truly […] all I can give her is the place in my memory I keep for her" (De Cervantes, 1605/1615, p. 790).

The only unwavering thought that remains is that Sancho must whip himself to disenchant Dulcinea. What can we do? Turn to the pastoral genre once again:

> As mankind, breathless, perseveres
> In tasks of vain frivolity,
> March, laughing through her shower-tears,
> Prepares spring's coming, secretly.
>
> (Gautier, 1852, p. 54)

Like Théophile Gautier, Don Quixote opts for this solution.

Regenerating language

What is left of the innocent life of shepherds? Only an unrepentant poet. Despite the lesson learned from the encounter with the bulls, Don Quixote starts to long, once again, for the life of a wanderer, and to dream of inventing a new world, like a child. But this time, the pastoral idyll is to be taken as a playground. To avoid confusing the imaginary with reality, a transitional space (Winnicott, 1971) of safety is provided for their forced retirement:

> This is the meadow where we came upon those gay shepherdesses and gallant shepherds who were trying to revive and imitate the pastoral Arcadia there […], in emulation whereof, if so be thou dost approve of it, Sancho, I would have ourselves turn shepherds, at any rate for the time I have to live in retirement. I will buy some ewes […] and, I under the name of the shepherd Quixotize and thou as the shepherd Panzino, we will roam the woods and groves and meadows singing songs here, lamenting in elegies there …
>
> (De Cervantes, 1605/1615, p. 791)

The mood is the conditional used by children when they play.

The place is the same, the same words and phrases are spoken, but the tone is different. When Dulcinea falls, like the *psyche* circling around the Real in Plato's dialogue *Phaedrus*, her wings are all creased, while one of her horses stumbles and throws her to the ground. What is left, Cervantes suggests, is the pastoral again, not as nostalgia for a golden age, but as the welcoming of a mother tongue, to revive a world where time has been regained.

In the very spot where they had been trampled on by a herd of bulls—Eugene Ionesco's totalitarian rhinoceros (1959)—Don Quixote will not imitate Arcadia, but create sheer poetry. At the edge of the forest, where animals, rocks, and trees, as well as fay creatures and fairies, speak to those we call "cracked", the two would-be shepherds transform voices and visions into joyful words, music, and rythms, resembling children's rhymes and revelry:

> I love the mountains
> I love the rolling hills
> I love the flowers
> I love the daffodils,
>   Boom-dee-a-da
>   Boom-dee-a-da
>   Boom-dee-yey
>   Boom-dee- yey
> I love the fireside
> When all the lights are low,
>   Boom-dee-a-da
>   Boom-dee-a-yey.

Through the gap opened by the announced loss of Dulcinea, and through the "gateless barrier" (Huikai, 1991) of the sheep pens, a multitude of new words emerge, creating a plural body of communion with nature:

> The oaks will yield us their sweet fruit with bountiful hand, the trunks of the hard cork trees a seat, the willows shade, the roses perfume, the widespread meadows carpets tinted with a thousand dyes; the clear pure air will give us breath, the moon and stars lighten the darkness of the night for us, songs shall be our delight, lamenting our joy, Apollo will supply us with verses, and love with

> conceits whereby we shall make ourselves famed for ever, not only in this but in ages to come.
>
> (De Cervantes, 1605/1615, p. 791)

And Don Quixote is right. In the summer, the mountains give away the perfume of their pastures and of the Nigritella, the lilac of fireweed, the yellow of bitterwort, the violet of gentians, the whistling alert of the Alpine marmot—and regenerate exhausted souls.

A new life begins, as a prelude to separation from Dulcinea. Silly nicknames are invented, which keep Don Quixote's caregivers at bay. Sanson Carrasco will be called "Samsonino", Nicholas the barber "Niculoso", and the curate "Curiambro", and there will be a shepherdess for each of them: "For the shepherdess whose lovers we shall be, we can pick names as we would pears."

Sancho will be quite happy to call his wife "Teresona".

And since Cervantes has not authorised his son to sail to Algeria, Don Quixote will content himself with the Arabic words that entered the Spanish language, Morisco words starting with *al-* or ending in *i-*: "It will be of great assistance to us in the perfect practice of this calling that I am something of a poet" (De Cervantes, 1605/1615, p. 792).

The "tarantula of poetry"—the spider that gives delusions and makes people dance the tarantella—also bites Carrasco, the barber and the curate, who join the pastoral choir in which the knight "will bewail [his] separation" and the others "will figure as [...] whatever may please [them] best" (De Cervantes, 1605/1615, p. 792). Sancho continues to daydream, imagining the beautiful wooden spoons he will carve while waiting for his daughter Sanchica to bring their dinner.

"But stay—[...] shepherds there are with more mischief than simplicity in them; I would not have her 'come for wool and go back shorn'; [...] and 'better a clear escape than good men's prayers'." A string of proverbs follows, to which Don Quixote tries to put an end by producing some of his own: "but it seems to me it is only 'preaching in the desert'; 'my mother beats me and I go on with my tricks'" (De Cervantes, 1605/1615, p. 793).

Not to be outdone, Sancho answers with another proverb: "The frying pan calling the kettle black."

Now, the knight proves his mastery in the art of proverbs and even presents a theory on their optimal use, similar to Jean Paulhan's remarks on the proverbs in Madagascar, saying, after several failed attempts: "[Now] when I quote them they fit like a ring to the finger." Likewise, Don Quichotte concludes that of these "short maxims drawn from the experience and observation of our wise men of old [...] the proverb that is not to the purpose is a piece of nonsense and not a maxim" (De Cervantes, 1605/1615, p. 793).

The astuteness of their exchange also echoes Socrates' analysis in the *Theaetetus*, according to which the intertwining of primary random elements, *stoicheia aloga* (Plato, c. 369 BC)—thoughts without a thinker, words taken for things, surviving voices or visions—produces the *logos*—speech and reason—to oppose the attack on the symbolic order, perpetrated by perversion. The mission with which Cervantes has entrusted us in the the Author's Preface is now clear.

Little by little

Acquiring access to the *logos* and becoming a subject in the chain of signifiers by disenchanting Dulcinea is one and the same thing. The Lady of one's thoughts has made it possible for the "thoughts without a thinker" (Bion, 1997) stemming from trauma to find an addressee, so that they could be thought. Now, "the unconscious structured like a language" (Lacan, 2003) has replaced the cut-away unconscious, made up of images of words and things having survived erasure. The agency of the Lady is gradually replaced by an agency of trust, a reliability impossible to imagine previously.

But what seems simple in theory is not so easy to put into practice, judging by the very long time the author needed to lead his heroes to this achievement. Now the pastoral idyll becomes really playful, and Sancho will soon get the idea of acquitting himself of the required whipping by flogging trees. "I should play-act fear", Wittgenstein was to say (1953). But this ruse has to be postponed. For the moment, he must bring Don Quixote to the "royal road" of dreams, as Freud was to call the main access to the repressed unconscious.

For the daydream of pastoral life did not appease the knight bereft of his Dulcinea. "They turned aside, and supped late and poorly", in Sancho's opinion. "Don Quixote obeyed nature so far as to sleep his first sleep, but did not give way to the second." He woke up his squire "to share the sufferings and feel the sorrows of [his master], if it be only for the sake of appearances" (De Cervantes, 1605/1615, p. 794).

Sancho's answer praises the symbolic value of dreams. Sleep, he says, is "the cloak that covers over all a man's thoughts [...], the universal coin wherewith everything is bought, [...] that makes the shepherd equal with the king and the fool with the wise man" (De Cervantes, 1605/1615, p. 795).

Here, their talking cure takes a turn towards the sphere of desire. When an analysis reaches this point, after a period of delusion or withdrawal, the analyst is happy. Now that the analysis seems to progress in a more orthodox way, beyond the primary process, it can advance more serenely toward the interpretation of dreams, with benevolent neutrality, free association, and symbolic echoes from the repressed unconscious. "Not at all!", the analyst is warned by Cervantes, who is all too familiar with reversals of fate. Now the unspeakable Real comes back in the form of a grunting drove of pigs which "came on in a surging mass, and without showing any respect for [their] dignity, passed right over the pair of them" (De Cervantes, 1605/1615, p. 795).

"I hate the common crowd and keep them at a distance" (Horace, 23 BC), said Horace. Although he has attempted to avoid the common crowd, Don Quixote is once again assailed by "unclean beasts" which cause "packsaddle, armor, Dapple and Rocinante [to be] left scattered on the ground and Sancho and [himself] at their wit's end".

This time, the knight's reaction is slightly different. *Bis repetita non placent*! (Repetitions are not well received). He doesn't react to the pigs the same way he reacted to the bulls, and takes responsibility for what happens. The reader becomes aware that through small brush-strokes, like those of the Impressionists, a barely visible displacement is brought about, which, in the end, produces an enormous change. It is as if the famous "domino effect" has worked backwards. By standing up, one of them makes all the other fallen dominos rise again.

Similarly, Robert Musil's remark: "[War] arises (like crime) from all those things that people ordinarily allow to dissipate in small irregularities" (1995, p. 1756) can also be inverted when a subject no longer allows himself to be the passive agent of the mob.

All he has to do is say no. And this is exactly the knight's attitude when confronted with the grumbling crowd, the same as Cervantes' attitude towards the pigs who shamelessly dismantled his quixotic work. The knight claims that "this insult is the penalty of [his] sin", for he had failed to defend Dulcinea. Deprived of the *hubris* that made him feel invincible, he now admits that he will die like everyone else, and composes a little madrigal to express the thoughts that fill his sleepless nights, singing "propped up against the trunk of a beech or a cork tree":

> When in my mind
> I muse, O Love, upon thy cruelty,
> To death I flee,
> In hope therein the end of all to find.
> But drawing near
> That welcome haven in my sea of woe,
> Such joy I know,
> That life revives, and still I linger here.
> Thus life doth slay,
> And death again to life restoreth me;
> Strange destiny,
> That deals with life and death as with play!
>
> (De Cervantes, 1605/1615, p. 796)

Much has happened since the mechanical production of such oxymorons by the Distressed Duena. While he sings, the knight sheds bitter tears because Dulcinea, who has been his whole life, is now fading away. Just as Psyche, after the departure of Eros, had to visit the Hades to experience her mortality, the knight now experiences his finitude. And Cervantes "[maintains] a strange silence" during the ensuing episode. Now the message we must pass on to the forger becomes clear.

In fact, this message had been illustrated, while we were finishing the writing of our book, by the following delusional episode.

CHAPTER SIX

Post-scriptum

Before submitting this manuscript to the publisher, I asked myself whether I should add another chapter. Gazing into dark, indistinct corners, I see a small toy box, and I hear the barking of Mirka, my Uncle Jean's dog.

The long-forgotten little box brings back the familiar sound of the gold-coloured screws and bolts of my Meccano sets, which sends me sailing toward unknown shores, like Magellan around Cape Horn in 1519.

7 March 2011

After several months of chemotherapy, the decision is made to perform major surgery to treat a bad case of stomach cancer. Six days after the operation, an infection makes a second surgery unavoidable. At this point, I veer off from the sequence of medical procedures.

The next day, I wake up somewhere in an airport. My hands and feet are bolted in place with the screws and bolts of the Meccano set. No doubt, this has something to do with the real restraints used in the intensive care unit, with a dangerously high fever, and with the drugs used to control post-operative pain.

In any case, for the moment I am pinned down, bolted to the little wooden box, with no consideration for my most elemental and private physical needs.

I scream. After a while, I hear someone asking if I know where I am. What I know is that a standard hospital clock, with a blue frame, will keep time during my entire stay in this one room. When I am asked: "Where are you?", I have learned to give the expected answer: "We are at the Cochin Hospital in Paris", although I have travelled thousands of kilometres, and have been gone hundreds of hours—which explains my exhaustion.

The clock of madness shows the same time over the entire territory, although space becomes distorted when I pass in just a few moments from one corridor to another for scan exams, thus being transported instantly from Paris to Provence, while the hospital clock remains my only objective reference point.

In the meantime, I am still pinned to my bed, unable to move. On the far-off banks of literature, I see Don Quixote. Hail, brother! In the midst of the disorder and violence, the calm voice of a doctor succeeds in explaining the ins and outs of my immobility. Three weeks later, when I was coming out of this episode, I recognised this voice in the surrounding hubbub, when by chance this same doctor was on call. I had felt right away that I could trust him, and now the ties that bound my hands and feet began to loosen.

I can now safely return to the toy box: its sliding cover is easy to move back and forth. For a few hours, or a few days, I am unaware that I can play with this open/close movement. There is also room for terror, when I spend a whole night certain that fire is raging all around my room. When the nurse answers my call, she reassures me, somewhat mockingly: "You know, Sir, this is a hospital. There are security systems everywhere; if there was a fire, dozens of sirens would go off." But in fact, the only thing I find slightly reassuring is the actual rain coming down in buckets outside.

The next night, less terrifying but more fantastical than the previous one, I take part, with pleasure and faith, in a fertility ritual. First, there is the creation of the tiny cavity where the seed will germinate, then a visit to the bowels of the earth by riding down steep stairs in a car.

Some shapes, like the packaging of the bandages, seem to smile at me sympathetically when, every three hours, someone comes to lift off Don Quixote's shield and take my temperature. In fact, the metal cap of the ear thermometer really looks like a helmet. At night, giant envelopes appear on the nurses' desk—probably my file, fantastic mail addressed to me, that I am not allowed to read. When daylight comes, all this disappears.

I have confidence in the fertility rite, because the previous year I had bought a pamphlet that described it minute by minute, in the village where I am now. Of course, this pamphlet does not exist. But I have faith. These people regenerate life.

And then, little by little, the simplicity of small things becomes comforting. Hour by hour, fewer problems, fewer complications, make it possible to foresee some safety. Only then can I imagine a back-and-forth flow between desire and reality.

There was *hubris* in confronting the Moirai. Yes, a violent confrontation with death took place.

In another toy box, much bigger this time, I will have to set out its components and its proper use in these circumstances.

The little box was there to tell me, after almost sixty-five years, that I would now have to write about all this as an essential part of my work as an analyst, far from the description of the effects of morphine or the distortions of thought in states of high fever.

Clearly, Don Quixote opened the transferential passage leading to the exploration of spaces, rhythms, and potential speech, which allow the analyst to travel down the road that is his own.

In the small toy box, and in the big one as well, books, verses, and shapes constitute the master key without which these experiences would be merely diagrams.

On my bookshelf, a few books stand on guard: Rabelais, Vassili Grossman, Hannah Arendt, *The Man without Qualities*, speaking of madness, war, and politics. The magnificent pages written by Robert Musil on the day of his death, under the heading "Breath of a Summer Day", open the way and protect me at the same time.

At this point in my life, I also have at my disposal an instrument that is just as delicate, which will start again the rhythm of breath and speech, like in the beginning of the *Ramayana* (Valmiki, 2000). Instead of having recourse to explanations and simplifications, it allows me, first of all, to establish areas of safety. Sparsely populated, their horizons and their forms are determined by the strength of the process.

Death is not very far; neither is life. My role consists only of reinforcing this distance step by step, in accordance with my means.

First, create breaths that are very short, even when pain is absent—small circles of air that multiply with regularity, where the will is already present. Ultimately, these achievments are related to the purification of the memories attached to them. Until, perhaps, it becomes possible to attain small parcels of pure time, of fluid sensations, places from which it would be good to see and to feel the flutter and gentle force of the breath of spring.

Not weighed down by memories, dates, or vivid colours, the rhythm of the breath has become independent of conscious effort. Books and poetry (strangely, not music) sustain the back-and-forth flow.

I can now let Don Quixote live out his destiny. I know that he and others wait for me and that we are in resonance, after this experience that is now part of my work and my life. Between two worlds, the heart and the breath ensure continuity.

Cochin Hospital in Paris, third week of April, 2011

Toying with hate

When Don Quixote and Sancho are kidnapped, this time not at sea, but deep in the countryside, by "some ten men on horseback and four or five on foot", in the same "strange silence" that reigned when Don Quixote had been carried away in a cage, they are assailed with insults in a language Sancho does not understand, and Don Quixote is petrified. He cannot make out what is happening to them, until he recognises the castle they had decided to leave a little earlier.

In the courtyard, under the watchful eye of the duke and duchess, the scene awaiting them is worthy of the Inquisition. In the centre, on a catafalque, lies the dead body of a young maiden, under the light of hundreds of torches and lamps. Sancho is clad in the robe of those condemned to the stake, painted with devils in the flames. On his head, they place the San Benito, a cardboard mitre also worn by repentants, who were hanged before being burned at the stake. He is warned not to speak, or he will be gagged. But despite all this, the ability to step back, acquired on the occasion of their first escape, manifests itself once again: "Don Quixote surveyed him too, and though fear had got the better of his faculties, he could not help smiling to see the figure Sancho presented" (De Cervantes, 1605/1615, p. 799).

In the profound silence, "for the silence itself kept silent", a handsome youth in a Roman habit sang a poem he had composed himself.

Don Quixote kept his thoughts to himself, but suspected a hoax. The message was clear. Altisidora, on the catafalque, has succumbed to the knight's cruelty, and Sancho must be tortured to restore her to life. But to no avail. Neither the knight nor the squire can be forced to feel guilty.

Slaps to the face, pinpricks to the body, and pinches to the arms delivered by "duenas with spectacles" make Sancho bellow like a bull: "I'll bear all in patience to serve these gentlefolk; but I won't let duenas touch me, though the devil should carry me off" (De Cervantes, 1605/1615, p. 800).

So saying, he attacks his tormentors, a lighted torch in his hand. At this point, Altisidora pretends to stir, to little effect on those present. The scene ends here … to be continued. But why invent this scenario worthy of the Marquis de Sade, just when everything seems to have been said?

The key to the mystery is provided by Cide Hamete, while the heroes sleep, this time in the same room. As a matter of fact, the bachelor Carrasco came back to see the duke and duchess after the page's visit to Sancho's village, to let them know about the recent duel, and help them to "[practise] this mystification" (De Cervantes, 1605/1615, p. 803). In case we should ever fall into such a trap, Cervantes gives us, through Cide Hamete, a talisman that will help us use our judgement: never forget that the perverse mechanism is stupid, even if its slyness is often taken for intelligence: "the duke and duchess were two fingers' breadth removed from being something like fools themselves when they took such pains to make game of a pair of fools".

It was in the same period that Ben Johnson declared: *The Devil Is an Ass* (1616). Or a pig, according to Cervantes, who clearly prefers donkeys to pigs and bulls. "A desert that exceeds every human imagination" (Allendesalazar, 2002, p. 183), St Teresa of Avila says about Hell, warning her nuns against the fascination with hellfire imagery. Indeed, Altisidora's intention when she bursts into Don Quixote's room is to enthrall him with one last seduction plot, modelled on the previous scene involving Duena Rodriguez. "Don Quixote […] huddled himself up and well nigh covered himself altogether with the sheets and counterpane of the bed […]. Altisidora seated herself on a chair at the head of the bed" (De Cervantes, 1605/1615, p. 804).

She intends to fascinate him with a sham *nekyia*, a visit to the underworld, complete with lurid illustrations of the Gates of Hell, "where some dozen or so of devils were playing tennis, all in breechs and doublets, with falling collars trimmed with Flemish bonelace", using books as tennis balls. In fact, one of the books, "a brand new" one, was that written by Avellaneda. Normally, the knight's heart should soften at the sight of this young girl, so touching and full of charm, and so eager to defend his cause: "and I, having heard them mention the name of Don Quixote whom I love and adore so, took care to retain this vision in my memory" (De Cervantes, 1605/1615, p. 805).

But Don Quixote responds with a return shot she can't intercept: "A vision it must have been, no doubt, for there is no other I in the world."

Like his father in the Preface, he now displays indifference.

Disenchantment

Don Quixote is no longer disposed to expose himself to blows, to flirt with fourteen-year-old damsels, or even to play the role of his father's hero. He has become who he is, thanks to all that he learned in the course of his adventures, which he in turn taught us.

"Become what you are", says Nietzsche, quoting Pindar. But he has shortened verse 72 of the *Second Pythian* written in the fifth century BC: "*Genoi oios essi mathon*" (Become what you are, once you have learned it).

The importance of learning is reasserted in two other verses of the *Third Phytian*, dedicated to Asklepios, the god of medicine: "*Me phila psucha*: My soul, do not seek eternal life, but exhaust the realm of the possible" (Pindar, c. 440–490 BC).

Earlier, Don Quixote would have leaped into the depths of hell to save the fair damsel. Even though the fake book-burning reminds him of the burning of his own library, he is now keeping at bay the phantoms of his father's traumatic revivals, and refuses to take on the puppet role assigned to him: "I am not disturbed by hearing that I am wandering in a fantastic shape in the darkness of the pit [...], for I am not the one that history treats of."

This reference to her fantastical tale causes the damsel to reveal the vulgarity of the proceedings. She calls him "soul of a mortar", and discloses the subterfuge: "All that you have seen tonight has been makebelieve; I'm not the woman to [...] suffer for such a camel, much less die!" (De Cervantes, 1605/1615, p. 805).

Don Quixote has put her in her place, after which he does the same thing to the young musician who has just entered his room: "Of a truth, [...], your worship has a most excellent voice; but [...] what have Garcilasso's stanzas to do with the death of his lady?"

The youth informs him that he is one of "the callow poets of our day [who] pilfer where [they choose]" (De Cervantes, 1605/1615, p. 806). A word to the wise! Not wanting to linger at the castle, Don Quixote makes his farewells again, advising Altisidora to employ herself making lace, since "lace is worn in hell" as well as on earth, instead of boring him with nonsense. Nothing much is left of the castle and of the events that took place there, except Sancho's flogging, on which the squire strives to shed the light of reason. Now Dulcinea's disenchantment is only a hair's breadth away.

After the torments suffered by his squire, Don Quixote agrees to pay for the lashes Sancho will inflict on himself to disenchant Dulcinea, as if they were closing a deal. Sancho decides to set a price for each lash, a price he increases when he sees that his master is inept in the art of negotiation. When the price reaches a quarter of a real, he takes the liberty to cheat and substitutes wood for the genuine currency of his buttocks. Trees will be used for the whipping. As he rips off their bark, he emits "such groans every now and then, that one would have thought at each of them his soul was being plucked up by the roots" (De Cervantes, 1605/1615, p. 810). The fulfilment of the quota of lashes has become a theatrical performance.

Now there is a separation between the spectators and the stage, between daydreaming and reality. Theoretically, all that remains is to unmask the fraud before the law, to be rid of it at last. This will be accomplished at "a hostelry which Don Quixote recognized as such and did not take to be a castle with moat, turrets, portcullis, and drawbridge" (De Cervantes, 1605/1615, p. 811). The walls were decorated with paintings showing Helen carried off by Paris, and Dido's despair after being abandoned by Aeneas. Seeing this, Sancho is prompted to predict: "I'll lay a bet that before long there won't be a tavern, roadside inn, hostelry, or barber's shop where the story of our doings won't be painted up."

Modern-day readers have seen this prediction borne out. Inspired by our own Dulcineas and by our travel agencies, we believe that all the inns in La Mancha are the very ones where the two heroes found shelter. And we marvel at seeing statues of the inseparable duo everywhere. Hearing Sancho's prediction, the knight is pleased to recognise its Quixotic tones: "Thou art a great philosopher, Sancho, thou speakest very sensibly; I know not who taught thee" (De Cervantes, 1605/1615, p. 786).

The squire confirms that he has had a good model. "Show me who your friends are and I'll tell you who you are." In all fairness, he also acknowledges Don Quixote's mastery of proverbs: "You chide me for uttering proverbs, and you string them in couples yourself."

This is what happens at the end of an analysis, when the patient and the analyst realise they have been changed by each other. At that point, fictional characters can mix with reality, without any danger to the psyche.

Testimony

Now, a character out of the forger's novel enters the inn; it is Don Alvaro Tarfe, whom Don Quixote questions, without revealing his own identity. Alvaro Tarfe asserts that Don Quixote "was a very great friend of [his]", to whom he "showed many kindnesses" and saved from many disasters. The knight then asks whether he himself bears any resemblance to Don Quixote, the hero of the novel. The answer is unequivocal: "No indeed, not a bit."

Alvaro Tarfe speaks with equal certainty about the squire, who is nothing like the one he has before him, for about the one in Avellanada's book, he observes: "I never heard him say anything that had any drollery in it."

At this point, Sancho lets the truth be known: "I am the real Sancho Panza, [...]. And the real Don Quixote of La Mancha [...] is the gentleman before you" (De Cervantes, 1605/1615, p. 814). And his argument is presented so cleverly, in such a convincing style, that the gentleman takes him at his word, needing no other proof.

Eventually, the knight learns that his fake counterpart has been "shut up in the Casa del Nuncio at Toldeo" (De Cervantes, 1605/1615, p. 814), like the young licentiate locked up in the Seville asylum, who must still be there after all these years. Now, Don Quixote can rise to the occasion and be, in the words of Mallarmé, "such as into Himself at last eternity changes him", when he learns, five hundred pages later, what a miserable fate he has escaped.

"I don't know whether I am good, but I can safely say I am not 'the Bad'."

Not altogether good, nor altogether bad—as they said in the Middle Ages—he has decided on his own not to go to Saragossa, refuted the false testimony, corrected the dates and place names, and above all, he will denounce the scoundrels to legal authorities who show up at the inn just in time:

> I am Don Quixote de La Mancha [...], and not the unlucky one that has attempted to usurp my name and deck himself out in my ideas. I entreat your worship [...] to be so good as to make a declaration before the *alcalde* of this village that you never in all your life saw me until now, and that neither am I the Don Quixote in print in the Second Part, nor this Sancho Panza, my squire, the one your worship knew.
>
> (De Cervantes, 1605/1615, p. 814)

When the sequels of trauma take perverse forms, the analysis always leads to a point of judgement where the analyst, witness to facts that have been denied until then, must take a stand against distortions of the truth. Thus, when Don Quixote frees himself from the lengthy confinement in which the forger attempted to hold him, he asks the character taken out of the same counterfeit pages to testify against the author who created him, and to publish the unequivocal truth. Don Alvaro pledges his word: "again I say and declare that what I saw I cannot have seen, and that what happened me cannot have happened".

This formulation cancels all possibility of falsification, and testifies to the truth before a legal authority. What a difference from the First Part, where the knight found himself in a "brawl with officers of the Holy Brotherhood" (De Cervantes, 1605/1615, p. 342)! Now, for the first time in the novel, the representative of the law carries out his function. After dinner, "The *alcalde* of the village came by chance into the inn together with a notary, and Don Quixote laid a petition before him, showing that it was requisite for his rights that Don Alvaro Tarfe, [...], should make a declaration before him" (De Cervantes, 1605/1615, p. 815). An official document is therefore drawn up in due form, stating that "the gentleman there present [declares] that he was not the one that was in print in a history entitled 'Second Part of Don Quixote of La Mancha, by one Avellaneda of Tordesillas'".

Only then can Dulcinea's disenchantment take place, thanks to this act of inscription, and not at all to the lashes Sancho infícts on beech trees again the following night, in the woods where the two heroes sleep in the open. Count as he may the lashes from a distance, we understand well that Don Quixote's numbers carry little weight compared to the symbolic act validated by a third party.

Cervantes insists on the fact that a perverse pact must never be respected, and that the scoundrel who usurps the agency of the law deserves to be paid back in kind. Often, the child in the abused adult continues to whip himself in order to excuse his tormentor and accuse himself; until the analyst asserts that he is not that to which the pervert reduced him. Then, time immobilised by the attempted murder of one's soul can be set in motion again little by little: "Don Quixote and Sancho were in high delight, as if a declaration of the sort was of any great importance to them, and as if their words and deeds did not plainly show the difference between the two Don Quixotes and the two Sanchos."

This declaration, duly signed and endorsed before the mayor, is indeed of great importance. Don Quixote has clearly entered a domain where good faith no longer relies only on "words and deeds", but on "all the formalities required in such cases". Now, the agency of the law can replace the agency of the Lady. Dulcinea is no longer the sole safe harbour for his thoughts. She can be inscribed in memory and be left in the past, allowing forgetfulness.

Sancho, clearly a confirmed analyst, no longer pays any attention to his master's checking, even when the latter goes up to every peasant woman they meet to verify that she is not Dulcinea, "as he held it absolutely certain that Merlin's promises could not lie" (De Cervantes, 1605/1615, p. 816). At the sight of their village at the top of a hill, Sancho fell to his knees in a salute to his motherland: "Open thine eyes, longed-for home, and see how thy son Sancho Panza comes back to thee, if not very rich, very well whipped! Open thy arms and receive, too, thy son Don Quixote, who, if he comes vanquished by the arm of another, comes victor over himself, which, as himself has told me, is the greatest victory anyone can desire."

Now, all they have to do is start off in the village on the right foot.

Victor over himself

There can be no doubt: Sancho's salute to the land that gives you life, protects you, and envelops you for your eternal rest—this salute constitutes the final message to the reader.

Today, the idea of victory over oneself has lost it meaning, since this self is, on the contrary, the object of pampering, of rejuvenating treatments, of anti-everything therapy, of plastic surgery, and in its name we get rid of old things, old people, cumbersome children, and fools. What, then, could be the meaning of gaining victory over oneself?

Cervantes describes three stages of this process.

First stage

The first starts with two *kledônes*, taken from the animistic world. A hare pursued by hunters with their greyhounds comes flying "to take shelter and hide itself under Dapple". Then a phrase is repeated by children who are fighting over a cage holding a cricket: "Thou shalt never see it again as long as thou livest" (De Cervantes, 1605/1615, p. 817).

Don Quixote, the hunted hunter, identifies with the hare, and believes that these words are signs telling him he will never see Dulcinea again. But to give her up also means giving up the world whose guiding star she has been. "*Malum signum, malum signum*!", the knight prophesies with good reason, like the Delphic Pythia or, more likely, the Cumaean Sybil, who speaks in Latin.

Sancho tries to avert this fate by making interpretations: "let's take it for granted that this hare is Dulcinea, and these greyhounds chasing it the malignant enchanters who turned her into a country wench; she flies, and I catch her and put her into your worship's hands, and you hold her in your arms and cherish her; what [...] ill omen is there to be found here?" (De Cervantes, 1605/1615, p. 817).

As if Dulcinea had to be flattered! In truth, it is the knight who trembles like a hare, sensing that death is near. In order to ensure that the omens are "broken and destroyed", Sancho buys the cage with the cricket for his master, as if this gift could also restore his access to Dulcinea. But Don Quixote no longer takes words for things. In fact, Sancho uses the cricket cage as Wittgenstein used his beetle box, not to enclose a private meaning—in this case, Dulcinea—but as the starting point of the possibility of speech.

Wittgenstein argued:

> Suppose everyone had a box with something in it: we call it a "beetle". No one can look into anyone else's box, and everyone says

> that he knows what a beetle is only by looking at his beetle.—Here it would be quite possible for everyone to have something different in his box ... The thing in the box has no place in the language-game at all; not even as a something: for the box might even be empty.
>
> (Wittgenstein, 1953, Sec. 293)

Indeed, the agency of the Lady has never appeared to be so empty. But this emptiness encompasses a language game. It is not possible to know what the other has in his private mind box as long as this other has not revealed it by telling or showing what is inside. Similarly, another poet/scientist, Erwin Schrödinger, had a box that held a virtual cat, not better off than the hare, since he was closed in with a radioactive atom. As long as the box remains closed, no one knows if the cat is dead or alive.

In the same way, now that Don Quixote is in this intermediary state where he slowly allows the far-away Lady of his Thoughts to leave him, he does not know what will become of him until he is able to say it, and above all, until he finds someone to say it to. Who? We, the readers, of course. We now guess what Cervantes wanted to tell us at the beginning, when he kept silent, saying: "there's no need of making words about it".

In the meantime, Don Quixote gives the hare back to the hunters—who are no doubt intending to make stew—thereby indicating that his own path is taking him in a definite direction: "let us push on and go into our village".

The second stage of entering the village resembles the medieval Feast of the Ass, when the animal would enter Notre-Dame Cathedral wearing sacerdotal garb.

Second stage

The ass is clad in the penitent's robe and mitre, which Sancho had insisted on keeping. At the entrance of the village, "upon the green", they come upon "the curate and the bachelor Sanson Carrasco busy with their breviaries" (De Cervantes, 1605/1615, p. 818). Albeit on a different scale, this triumphant entrance emulates the heroes' arrival in Barcelona. The street urchins, "who are lynxes that nothing escapes"—and whom Murillo's paintings would soon make famous—came running to see them. Teresa Panza, "with her hair all loose and half naked", was dragging Sanchica by the hand; the girl has been waiting for her father "as for the showers of May". The heroes' welcoming committee was composed of the inevitable quartet—barber, curate, niece, and housekeeper—augmented to include the bachelor.

Each one soon went off to his own home, Sancho walking between his wife and daughter, who held him by the belt with one hand while she "led Dapple" with the other (De Cervantes, 1605/1615, p. 818). Sancho had brought money "got by [his] own industry without wronging anybody". Señora Panza is not impressed with this proclamation of integrity: "You bring the money, my good husband", said Teresa, "and no matter whether it was got this way or that; for, however you may have got it, you'll not have brought any new practice into the world".

For his part, Don Quixote lost no time before telling the bachelor and the curate about his defeat and his resolve to live a pastoral life. Using the conditional tense again to set the mood, he announced that "he would buy sheep [...]; and he besought them [...] to consent to be his companions [...], for he had given them names that would fit them to a T".

Sanson Carrasco jumps at the chance to be published at low cost, and reminds them of his talents as a poet, offering to write verses that would rhyme with all the names of current celebrities.

The housekeeper, "with fifty years upon [her] head", as she says, quickly intervened to interrupt the rejoicing. She is well acquainted with shepherds, and besides, she is not drunk. Her description of pastoral life can still be seen taking place today in mountain pastures during the summer: waking at dawn after a short night spent sleeping on planks, milking the sheep twice a day, making the cheese, dealing with lambing in adverse weather, watching out for birds of prey and wild beasts: "will your worship be able to bear, out in the fields, the heat of summer, and the chills of winter, and the howling of the wolves? Not you; for that's a life and a business for hardy men, bred and seasoned to such work almost from the time they were in swaddling clothes" (De Cervantes, 1605/1615, p. 820).

Raised for the profession of arms, Don Quixote admits that his duty does not lie in such work. He understands that the truth is to be sought elsewhere: "help me to bed, for I don't feel very well". On the verge of collapse, he does not fail those close to him: "knight-errant now or wandering shepherd to be, I shall never fail to have a care for your interests". Now he enters the final stage.

The death of Don Quixote

In Don Quixote's case, the final hour which no one can predict is announced in the grand style of the Ancients: "As nothing that is man's can last for ever, but all tends ever downward from its beginning to its end, and above all man's life […], its end and close came when he least looked for it."

The psychiatric diagnosis of Don Quixote's melancholia caused by his defeat does not hold true simply because we have all to die. When Providence—the Fates, the Norns, the Moirai, or the Parcae—decided to cut the thread of his life, "a fever settled upon him and kept him in his bed for six days, during which he was often visited by his friends, the curate, the bachelor, and the barber, while his good squire Sancho Panza never quit his bedside".

The three stages of grief: depression, anger, and acceptance, at the perspective of death, are exactly as Elisabeth Kübler-Ross described them (1970). Still, her interest in dying patients was regarded with suspicion, as if we had the right to refuse to die, unless death were caused by a medical error or by melancholy.

As is true for all of us on such occasions, guilt overwhelms Sancho, who blames himself for causing the knight's fatal fall by "not girthing Rocinante properly" (De Cervantes, 1605/1615, p. 823). Earlier, he has been trying, like the others, as we all do, to cheer up his master and encourage him to get well. Sanson Carrasco has already composed "an eclogue that would take the shine out of all Sannazaro had ever written, […]. But for all this Don Quixote could not shake off his sadness."

They all say what people say in such situations in order to avoid facing the dying man's detachment. Only the doctor they call in is definite in his assessment. After feeling his pulse, he told the knight that "it would be well for him to attend to the health of the soul, as that of his body was in a bad way" (De Cervantes, 1605/1615, p. 821). The doctor leans towards a psychological cause: he was of the opinion "that melancholy and depression were bringing him to his end". Fortunately, at the time there were no mood-enhancing drugs that would have allowed his patient to die in great shape. Once the diagnosis is official, the women begin to weep.

Lacking our postmodern remedies, Don Quixote remembered the old lessons of stoicism, and heard the doctor's words calmly. He then asked them "to leave him to himself, as he had a wish to sleep a little". He seemed to sink into a coma.

But the author who brought him into being has an excellent surprise in store for him: a mystical revelation which transforms the renunciation of his past life into the inheritence he has passed down to us.

Awakening

After having acquitted himself of his debt to his father by wiping out the stain—"*mancha*"—of war, slavery, and perversion, Don Quixote returns to his senses in a flash. When he awakens after six hours of sleep at one stretch, he cries out. The cry that inaugurates the trance in animistic cultures usually signals that a god or a spirit is taking hold of someone's soul. Here, this cry indicates that Don Quixote has recovered his soul.

"Blessed be Almighty God!"

The experience of awakening he describes to his niece resembles the *satori* in the Zen tradition. As St Teresa of Avila would put it, his soul has finally reached its abode, and "when it dwells there, it is inexorably a plural soul" (Allendesalazar, 2002, p. 196). The knight declares: "My reason is now free and clear, rid of the dark shadows of ignorance."

His rejection of the books he loved until now springs from a veritable conversion. He no longer needs to rely on visions of words and things—so crucial when the imaginary realm is destroyed—to confront "furies from who knows where", as Socrates says in the *Phaedrus*. Thus, he can throw away the books, and even "loathe them", since the cathartic process that served to cleanse his father's wounds is now completed (De Cervantes, 1605/1615, p. 822).

Similarly, the stunned analyst often realises that at the end of the psychanalytic path, the patient has forgotten, or repressed, all the patient interweaving achieved in the transference to escape anti-subjective traps. The traumatic memory of surviving images that show what cannot be said has been replaced by the memory of repression, which is able to forget, for it is articulated by symbolic inscriptions like the name engraved on a tomb.

Don Quixote's death, like that of Socrates in the *Phaedo*, prefigures Cervantes' last moments. He no longer needs the name by which he was known in combat and in slavery, Saavedra (Garcés, 2002, p. 185). Similarly, Don Quixote gives up his literary identity. Under that name, in the First Part of the novel, he won the battle against the erasure of Cervantes' experience of war and slavery, and he took up arms again, in the Second Part, against forgery.

His mission accomplished, he can assume his legal name, Alonso Quixano, written on his baptism certificate. The reader learns, after the hesitations in the first pages—"Quixada, Quesada…"—that he was called Alonso Quixano. Like the delusions woven by descendants from the untold histories of their ancestors, his "shrewd lunacies" (De Cervantes, 1605/1615, p. 399), in other words his *folly*, is more a device than a destiny.

Cervantes gives back the *Caballero ingenioso* his true identity. By doing so, he points out a remarkable characteristic of the treatment of madness and trauma. When Don Quixote wakes up with a clear mind, those around him take his words for another fit of madness, when in fact what they are witnessing is a complete return to his senses. Indeed, the prophetic style of his declaration is impressive: "Good news for you, good sirs, that I am no longer Don Quixote of la Mancha, but Alonso Quixano, whose way of life won for him the name of Good."

It is worth repeating that nothing resembles more the loss of one's senses than the return to them. Taking hold of this ingenious device and letting it go require the same energy. When the knight is "drawing near death", he finds himself in "extremities [where] man must not trifle with his soul".

In the stirrup

Two years later, on 23 April 1616, Cervantes reaches the same frontier. Like his hero, he is "filled with an ardent desire to live" (Allendesalazar, 2002, p. 222). Just when he is facing death, which he has approached so often, his desire to live is intense. Two weeks after taking his final vows as a member of the Tertiary Order of St Francis on 19 April 1616, he wrote, in the Dedication of *Persiles* to the Count of Lemos: "In the stirrup, with the agony of death upon me, great lord, I write to you. Yesterday they gave me extreme unction […]. The time is short, my pains are increasing, my hopes are diminishing; and yet, with it all, the desire I have to live keeps me alive" (De Cervantes, 1617).

In the same way, the curate receives Don Quixote's confession, while everyone sheds rivers of tears, and his author begins to compose his eulogy: under one identity or the other, he "was always of a gentle disposition and kindly in all his ways, and hence he was beloved, not only by those of his own house, but by all who knew him" (De Cervantes, 1605/1615, p. 823).

To describe him as "gentle"—"peaceful" in the French translation—seems paradoxical, unless we think of the Latin phrase *Si vis pacem, para bellum* (If you want peace, prepare for war), and consider his fight for the touchstone of truth as a fundamental element of peace.

Don Quixote's will brings to mind François Villon's poem "The Great Testament" (1489). To Sancho, he leaves all the money they had when they left the ducal castle, but above all, the acknowledgement *ad vitam eternam* of his exceptional candour and loyalty. When he asks his squire to forgive him for leading him "to seem as mad as myself", Sancho voices his despair at the prospect of losing him: "Ah! don't die, master, but take my advice and live many years; for the foolishest thing a man can do in this life is to let himself die without rhyme or reason, without anybody killing him, or any hands but melancholy's making an end of him" (De Cervantes, 1605/1615, p. 823).

Here, melancholy is not borne by the dying man, but by those who will mourn him. This commentary is addressed to all of us who try to convince the one who is dying to live a little longer to save us from grief. Elisabeth Kübler-Ross was incensed to see the lack of understanding shown to those who are serene in this passing. In the last hours of his life, Cervantes provided the reader with the same lesson in living, when his "desire to live [kept him] alive". "Sirs, not so fast", said Don Quixote, "'in last year's nests there are no birds this year'. I was mad, now I am in my senses [...]; and may my repentance and sincerity restore me to the esteem you used to have for me."

This reflection on madness, for which he takes complete responsibility, is the strength he passes on to his countless disciples.

After giving all his property to his niece, and bequeathing to his housekeeper all the wages he owed her, plus an additional sum for a gown, he entrusts us with a paradoxical message for the forger. Now, when he is in the process of forgiving those who have offended him, he is also asking their forgiveness. If, by chance, we should come upon the author who disguises his name, as we are told in the Author's Preface, our final mission is formulated by the knight with a last flash of humour: "that, if any happy chance should lead them to discover the author who is said to have written a history [...], they beg of him on my behalf as earnestly as they can to forgive me for having been [...] the cause of his writing so many and such monstrous absurdities" (De Cervantes, 1605/1615, p. 824).

Don Quixote's agony lasted three more days, during which the niece ate compulsively, the housekeeper drank likewise, and Sancho was full of cheer, "for inheriting property wipes out or softens down in the heir the feeling of grief". After he gave up the ghost, Cervantes had the curate add a codicil to the death certificate, stating that Don Quixote of La Mancha had indeed passed away, "in order to remove the possibility of any other author save Cide Hamete Benengeli bringing him to life again falsely and making interminable stories out of his achievements".

The soul and the pen

Here, the Moorish author brings his tale to an abrupt end, and speaks directly to his pen, which he has now put on the shelf: "Rest here, hung up by this brass wire [...], O my pen [...]; here shalt thou remain long ages hence, unless presumptuous or malignant storytellers take thee down to profane thee" (De Cervantes, 1605/1615, p. 825).

And to better protect it, he utters a magic formula: "Hold off! Ye weaklings; hold your hands!"

In a superb prosopopoeia, the pen answers, speaking the words the forger tried to steal from her. She is Don Quixote, the lost feather of the winged soul of Cervantes, reunited at last with his Dulcinea, literature, which did not let itself be deceived either.

> For me alone [*sola*] was Don Quixote born, and I for him; it was his to act, mine to write; we two together make but one, notwithstanding and in spite of that pretended Tordesillesque writer who has ventured [...] with his great, course ill-trimmed ostrich quill to write the achievements of my valiant knight.
>
> (De Cervantes, 1605/1615, p. 825)

Cervantes' testament hands down to us the will to always oppose the violation of our psyche or the work we create. Cide Hamete speaks on his behalf: "And I shall remain satisfied, and proud to have been the first [*el primero*] who has ever enjoyed the fruit of his writings" (De Cervantes, 1605/1615, p. 826).

For Don Quixote is Cervantes' soul, quill, and lance, the psychic device of madness without which he could not have inscribed the epic journey of his life, in the face of pre-planned erasure. It is now up to us, readers and analysts, to follow his example.

A word to the wise!

REFERENCES

Allen, W. (Dir.) (1985). *The Purple Rose of Cairo*.

Allendesalazar, M. (2001). *Thérèse d'Avila: deuxième autobiographie*. Paris: Berg International.

Allendesalazar, M. (2002a). Don Quichotte, livres, rêves et folie. *Études*, No. 3962.

Allendesalazar, M. (2002b). *Thérèse d'Avila, l'image au féminin*. Paris: Seuil.

Allendesalazar, M. (2004). Desengano. In: B. Cassin (Ed.), *Vocabulaire européen des philosophies*. Paris: Seuil.

Antisthenes (1992). *Les Ciniques grecs*. Ed. and Trans. L. Paquet (p. 67). Paris: Le Livre de Poche.

Apuleius (1999). *The Golden Ass, or Metamorphoses*. Trans. E. J. Kenney. London: Penguin Classics.

Arbousse-Bastide, P. (1972). Auguste Comte et la folie. Les Sciences de la folie. Les éditions de l'EHESS.

Arendt, H. (1951). *The Origins of Totalitarianism*. Cleveland: The World Publishing Company.

Arrabal, F. (1996). *Un escalavo llamado Cervantes* (A Slave Named Cervantes). Madrid: Espasa Calpe.

Aubailly, J.-C. (1984). *Le Monologue, le Dialogue et la Sottie*. Paris: Vrin.

Barker, P. (1992). *Regeneration*. London: Penguin Books.

Barrois, C. (1993). *Psychanalyse du guerrier*. Paris: Hachette.

Baudelaire, C. (2011). To the reader. In: W. Fowlie (Trans.), *The Flowers of Evil and Paris Spleen*. New York: Dover Thrift Editions.

Benedetti, G. (1998). *Le Sujet emprunté: Le vécu psychotique du patient et du thérapeute* (The Borrowed Subject: Symbiosis between Patient and Analyst). Toulouse: Érès.

Binswanger, L., & Warburg, A. (2007). *La Guérison infinie: Histoire clinique d'Aby Warbur*. Paris: Rivages.

Bion, W. R. (1961). *Experiences in Groups and Other Papers*. London: Tavistock.

Bion, W. R. (1967). *Second Thoughts*. London: William Heineman Medical Books.

Bion, W. R. (1982). *The Long Week-End (1897–1919)*. London: Karnac.

Bion, W. R. (1983). *Two Papers: Grid and Caesura*. London: Karnac.

Bion, W. R. (1997). *Taming Wild Thoughts*. London: Karnac.

Bosco, H. (1978). *Culotte the Donkey*. Oxford: Oxford University Press.

Braudel, F. (1949). *The Mediterranean and the Mediterranean World in the Age of Philip II*. Berkeley: University of California Press, 1995.

Bremmer, J., & Roodenburg, H. (Eds.) (1992). The rationale of gestures in the West. In: J.-C. Schmidt, *A Cultural History of Gesture*. New York: Cornell University Press.

Bruno, G. (1585). *The Heroic Frenzies* (Fourth Dialogue). Trans. P. E. Memmo. Chapel Hill: University of North Carolina Press, 1964.

Canavaggio, J. (1977). *Cervantes dramaturge: Un théâtre à naître*. Paris: PUF.

Canavaggio, J. (1991). *Cervantes*. New York: W. W. Norton.

Canavaggio, J. (2005). *Don Quichotte, du livre au mythe. Quatre siècles d'errance*. Paris: Fayard.

Cassou, J. (1949). *Don Quichotte*. Paris: Gallimard.

Cassou, J. (1953). *La Mémoire courte*. Paris: Mille et Une Nuit, 2001.

Caviness, M. (2003). Iconoclasm and iconophobia: four historical case studies. *Diogenes, 199*: 99–114.

Cazotte, J. (1772). *The Devil in Love*. London: Dedalus European Classics, 2011.

Coppola, F. F. (Dir.) (1972). *The Godfather*.

Countess de Ségur (2011). *Monsieur Cadichon: Memoires of a Donkey*. New York: Simon & Schuster.

D'Arras, J. (2013). *Le Roman de Mélusine* (1392–94). In: G. Knight, *The Book of Melusine of Lusignan*. London: Skylight Press.

Damasio, A. (2005). *Descartes' Error*. London: Penguin Books.

Davoine, F. (2016). *Don Quixote: Fighting Melancholia*. London: Karnac.

De Cervantes, M. (1585). *Galatea: A Pastoral Romance*. Trans. G. W. J. Gyll. London: Bell and Daldy, 1876; London: Forgotten Books, 2015.

De Cervantes, M. (1605/1615). *Don Quixote*. Trans. J. Ormsby. Canterbury: Canterbury Classics/Baker & Taylor, 2013.

De Cervantes, M. (1615). *Retablo de las maravillas* (The Marvellous Puppet Show). Oxford: Oxford University Playwriting and Dramaturgy Society (Trans.), 2016.

De Cervantes, M. (1617). *The Trials of Persiles y Sigismunda*. Trans. C. Weller & C. A. Colahan. Cambridge, MA: Hackett Classics, 2009.

De Lamartine, A. (1993). Loneliness. In: D. Hillery (Ed.), *The Meditations Poetiques*. Durham: Durham Modern Languages Series, University of Durham Press.

De Nerval, G. (1851). Artemis, and The Golden Lines. In: P. Joy (Trans.), *The Chimeras*. Vancouver: Anvil Press Poetry, 1984.

De Rojas, F. (1499). *Celestina*. Trans. P. Bush. London: Penguin Classics, 2009.

De Ronsard, P. (2002a). *Hymn to Demons*. London: Penguin Classics.

De Ronsard, P. (2002b). *Selected Poems*. London: Penguin Classics.

De Rotelande, H. (circa 1180). *Ipomadon*. Ed. R. Purdle. Oxford: Oxford University Press, 2001.

Desfossés, J., Jacques, A., & Prilaux, G. (2009). *Great War Archeology*. Paris: Éditions Ouest-France.

Diderot, D. (1776). *Rameau's Nephew*. Trans. Ian C. Johnston. Oxford: Benediction Classics, 2011.

Drury, M. O'C. (1981). Conversations with Wittgenstein. In: R. Rhees (Ed.), *Ludwig Wittgenstein: Personal Recollections*. Oxford: Blackwell Publishing.

D'Urfé, H. (1658). *Astrea: A Romance/Written in French by Messire Honore D'Urfe; and Translated by a Person of Quality*. Trans. J. Davies. London: Ecbo Editions, Proquest, 2001.

Erasmus, D. (2010). *The Praise of Folly*. Trans. J. Wilson. London: Aeterna Publishing.

Faulkner, W. (1936). *Absalon, Absalon*. New York: Random House, 1990.

Felman, S. (2002). *The Juridical Unconscious*. Cambridge, MA: Harvard University Press.

Flacelière, R. (1966). *Greek Oracles*. London: Paul Elek.

Freud, S. (1895). Project for a scientific psychology. *S. E., 1*: 281–397. London: Hogarth.

Freud, S. (1919). The uncanny. *S. E., 17*: 217–252. London: Hogarth.

Garcés, M. A. (2002). Writing Algiers: masters, slaves and renegades, books and manuscripts in the Ottoman Empire. In: *Cervantes in Algiers: A Captive's Tale* (pp. 66–123). Nashville: Vanderbilt University Press.

Gautier, T. (1852). Spring's first smile. In: *Théophile Gautier: Selected Lyrics*. Trans. N. R. Shapiro. New Haven: Yale University Press, 2012.

Giraldi, G. A. (1998). *Riche journal d'un artiste pauvre: Le carnet des campagnes d'un sculpteur d'églises baroques en Savoie*. Montmélian, Savoie: La Fontaine de Siloé.

Gouhier, H. (1997). *La Vie d'Auguste Comte*. Paris: Vrin.

Greenberg, J. (1989). *I Never Promised You a Rose Garden*. New York: American Library.

Herrigel, E. (1999). *Zen in the Art of Archery*. London: Vintage.

Homer (8th century BC). *The Odyssey*. Trans. R. Fagles. London: Penguin Classics, 1999.

Horace (23 BC). *The Odes* (Book III). Princeton, NJ: Princeton University Press, 2005.

Hugo, V. (1856). Continuation. In: E. H. Blackmore & A. M. Blackmore (Trans.), *Selected Poems of Victor Hugo: A Bilingual Edition*. Chicago: University of Chicago Press, 2004.

Hugo, V. (1859). *The Legend of the Centuries*. London: G. W. Dillingham, 1894.

Huikai, W. (1991). *The Gateless Barrier*. Trans. R. Aitken. New York: North Point Press.

Ionesco, E. (1994). *Rhinoceros and Other Plays*. London: Grove Press.

Izutsu, T. (2001). *Toward a Philosophy of Zen Buddhism*. Boulder, CO: Shambhala.

Jammes, F. (1898). From morning Angelus to evening Angelus. In: *Selected Poems of Francis Jammes*. Logan, UT: Utah State University Press, 1976.

Jarry, A. (1896). *Ubu Roi*. New York: Dover Publications, 2003.

Jéquier, C. (1993). Portrait du fou avec gourdin et fromage (Portrait of fool with coudgel and cheese). *Paragone*, August.

Jéquier, C. (2001). *La Folie, un péché médieval*. Paris: L'Harmattan.

Johnson, B. (1616). *The Devil is an Ass, and Other Plays*. Oxford: Oxford University Press, 2000.

Kafka, F. (1915). *The Metamorphosis*. Trans. I. Johnston. The Kafka Project, 2003.

Kafka, F. (1919). *In the Penal Colony*. London: Penguin Classics, 2011.

Kafka, F. (1925). *Diaries, 1910–1923*. New York: The Schocken Kafka Library, 1988.

Kübler-Ross, E. (1970). *On Death and Dying*. New York: Macmillan.

La Boétie, É. (1548). *Discourse on Voluntary Servitude*. Trans. H. Kurtz. Columbia: Columbia University Press, 1942.

Lacan, J. (1975). *Encore: The Seminar of Jacques Lacan* (Book XX, 1972–73). New York: W. W. Norton.

Lacan, J. (1997). *The Seminar of Jacques Lacan: The Ethics of Psychoanalysis* (Book VII), London: W. W. Norton.

Lacan, J. (2001f). Seminar XVII: *Psychoanalysis Upside Down: The Reverse Side of Psychoanalysis, 1969–1970*. Trans. C. Gallagher, unpublished.

Lacan, J. (2003). *Écrits: A Selection*. Trans. B. Fink. London: W. W. Norton, 2007.

Larned, W. T. (1925). *Reynard the Fox and Other Fables*. Chicago: Volland.

Laub, D. (1992). Bearing witness, or the vicissitudes of listening. In: S. Felman & D. Laub (Eds.), *Testimony*. London: Routledge.

Le Goff, J. (1986). *The Birth of Purgatory*. Trans. A. Goldhammer. Chicago: University of Chicago Press.

Le Goff, J. (2009). *Saint Louis*. Indiana: University of Notre Dame Press.

Le Goff, J., & Schmitt, J.-C. (1984). Le Charivari (Mystical bedlam, madness, anxiety and healing in seventeenth-century England). *Économies, Sociétés, Civilisations*, 1.

Levergeois, B. (1995). *Giordano Bruno*. Paris: Fayard.

Lin Tsi (AD 867). In: K. Nukariya (Trans.), *The Religion of the Samurai*. The Library of Alexandria, 1984.

Lope de Vega, F. (1618). *Fuenteovejuna*. Trans. S. Applebaum. New York: Dover Publications (Dual Language), 2012.

Losey, J. (Dir.) (1963). *The Servant*.

Marrast, R. (Ed.) (1983). *Théâtre espagnol du XVIe siècle*. Paris: Gallimard.

McGuire, W. (Ed.) (1974). *Freud–Jung Letters*. London: Routledge.

Melville, H. (1891). *Billy Bud, Sailor*. London: Penguin Classics, 1985.

Michelet, J. (1957). *Joan of Arc*. Michigan: University of Michigan Press.

Mishima, Y. (1959). *The Temple of the Golden Pavilion*. Trans. J. Morris. Avon: Harper Collins.

Molière (2004). *The Miser and Other Plays*. London: Penguin Classics.

Musil, R. (1995). *The Man without Qualities* (Vol. II). Trans. S. Wilkins & B. Pike. New York: Alfred A. Knopf.

Nagy, G. (1979). *The Best of the Achaens*. Baltimore: The Johns Hopkins University Press.

Nasar, S. (1998). *A Beautiful Mind*. New York: Simon & Schuster.

Neilli, R. (1974). *L'Érotique des troubadours*, Vol. 1. Paris: Union générale d'éditions.

Ordine, N. (1996). *Giordano Bruno and the Philosophy of the Ass*. Trans. H. Baranski. New Haven: Yale University Press.

Orwell, G. (1950). *Nineteen Eighty-Four*. London: Penguin, 2008.

Ovid (AD 8). *The Metamorphoses*. Trans. A. Mandelbaum. New York: Harcourt Brace, 1995. [Also Trans. A. S. Kline, *Poetry in Translation*, Book II, 2000.]

Paulhan, J. (1993). *L'Expérience du proverb*. Paris: L'Échoppe.

Pindar (c. 440–490 BC). *The Odes* (Pythian III, verses 61, 62). Trans. C. M. Bowra. London: Penguin Classics, 1982.

Plato (c. 385–370 BC). *Symposium*. Edinburgh: CreateSpace, 2013.
Plato (380 BC). *The Republic*. Edinburgh: Black & White Classics, 2014.
Plato (c. 370 BC). *Phaedrus*. Trans. S. Scully. Massachusetts: Focus Philosophical Library, 2003.
Plato (c. 369 BC). *Theaetetus*. Trans. B. Jowett. New York: The Liberal Arts Press, 1955.
Proust, M. (1927). *Time Regained*. Final volume of *Remembrance of Things Past*. New York: Modern Library, 1999.
Rabelais, F. (c. 1532–1564). *Gargantua and Pantagruel*. London: Penguin Classics, 2006.
Racamier, P.-C. (1992). *Le génie des origines: Psychanalyse et psychose*. Paris: Payot.
Ravel, M. (1925). *The Child and the Spells*, fantasy ballet with libretto by Colette. [He also composed *Don Quixote and Dulcinea* (1932); libretto in verse by Paul Morand.]
Renou, L. (1972). *Religions of Ancient India*. Delhi: South Asia Books.
Roditi, E. (1986). *A Glimpse of Robert Musil. BOMB Magazine* (winter).
Roggers and Hammerstein (1965). *The Sound of Music* (Broadway show).
Rossellini, R. (Dir.) (1950). *The Flowers of St. Francis*.
Rousset, D. (1948). *Le pitre ne rit pas*. Paris: Éditions du Pavois.
St John of the Cross (1585). *A Spiritual Canticle*. Trans. D. Lewis. New York: Cosimo Classics, 2007.
Saviano, R. (2008). *Gomorrah*. London: Pan Books.
Schmitt, J.-C. (1999). *Ghosts in the Middle Ages*. Trans. T. L. Fagan. Chicago: University of Chicago Press.
Shakespeare, W. (c. 1599–1602). *Hamlet*. New York: Dover Thrift Editions, 1992.
Stein, R. (2010). Notes on mind control: the malevolent uses of emotion as a dark mirror of the therapeutic process. In: A. Harris & S. Botticelli (Eds.), *First, Do No Harm* (pp. 251–277). New York: Routledge.
Sterne, L. (1999). *The Life and Opinions of Tristram Shandy, Gentleman*. London: Wordsworth Editions.
Swift, J. (1704). Digression on madness. In: *A Tale of a Tub*. New York: Serenity Publishers, 2011.
Swift, J. (1711). *A Meditation upon a Broomstick*. New York: Nabu Press, 2011.
Valmiki (2000). *Ramayana*. Trans. W. Buck. Delhi: Mortilal Banarsidass.
Vilar, P. (1971). The age of Don Quixote. *New Left Review, I (68)*.
Villon, F. (1489a). Ballad of Dead Ladies. Trans. D. G. Rossetti. In: *Ballads Done into English from the French of François Villon*. Portland, ME: Thomas B. Mosher, 1904.

Villon, F. (1489b). Les Regrets de la Belle Heaulmière. In: J. Dufournet (Ed.), *Poésies*. Paris: Garnier-Flammarion, 1992.

Villon, F. (1489c). The Ballad of Proverbs. *The World's Wit and Humour*, Vol. X, 1906.

Virgil (c. 29 BC). *The Georgics* (Book 4). New York: Nabu Press, 2012.

Von Kleist, H. (2004). *Heinrich von Kleist: Selected Writings*. Trans. D. Constantine. Indianapolis: Hackett Publishing.

Walser, R. (1908). *The Assistant*. Trans. S. Bernofsky. *New Directions*, 2007.

Warburg, A. (1923a). A lecture on serpent ritual.Trans. W. F. Mainland. *Journal of the Warburg Institute*, 2(14): 1938–1939.

Warburg, A. (1923b). A lecture on serpent ritual. Trans. W. F. Mainland. *Journal of the Warburg Institute*, *4*, April 1939: 277–292.

Warburg, A. (1925). "L'art du portrait et de la bourgeoisie florentine" (The Art of Portraiture and the Florentine Bourgeoisie). In: *Essais Florentins*. Paris: Hazan, 2015.

Winnicott, D. W. (1971). *Playing and Reality*. London: Routledge Classics.

Wittgenstein, L. (1929). *A Lecture on Ethics*. London: John Wiley & Sons, 2014.

Wittgenstein, L. (1934–1936). Notes for lectures on "private experience" and "sense data". *The Psychological Review, 77(3)* (July 1968).

Wittgenstein, L. (1953). *Philosophical Investigations*. Trans. G. Ascombe. Oxford: Oxford University Press, 1983.

Wittgenstein, L. (1966). Conversations on Freud. In: *Lectures and Conversations on Aesthetics, Psychology and Religious Belief*. Oxford: Blackwell.

Wittgenstein, L. (1967). *Remarks on Frazer's Golden Bough*. Trans. J. Beversluis. In: C. G. Luckhardt (Ed.), *Wittgenstein, Sources and Perspectives*. New York: Cornell University Press, 1979.

Xingjian, G. (2000). Nobel Lecture. Nobelprize.org.

INDEX